Professional Communication in Speech-Language Pathology

How to Write, Talk, and Act Like a Clinician

Third Edition

A. Embry Burrus
Laura B. Willis

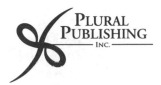

PLURAL
PUBLISHING
INC.

PLURAL PUBLISHING
INC.

5521 Ruffin Road
San Diego, CA 92123

e-mail: info@pluralpublishing.com
Website: http://www.pluralpublishing.com

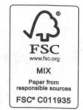

Library of Congress Cataloging-in-Publication Data

Names: Burrus, A. Embry, author. | Willis, Laura B., author.
Title: Professional communication in speech-language pathology : how to write, talk, and act like a clinician / A. Embry Burrus, Laura B. Willis.
Description: Third edition. | San Diego, CA : Plural Publishing, [2017] | Includes bibliographical references and index.
Identifiers: LCCN 2016013825| ISBN 9781597567244 (alk. paper) | ISBN 1597567248 (alk. paper)
Subjects: | MESH: Speech-Language Pathology--education | Clinical Competence | Interpersonal Relations | Professional Practice
Classification: LCC RC428.5 | NLM WL 18 | DDC 616.85/5—dc23
LC record available at http://lccn.loc.gov/2016013825

Professional Communication in Speech-Language Pathology

How to Write, Talk, and Act Like a Clinician

Third Edition

CONTENTS

PREFACE

> It was 8:14 on Monday morning and Abby strolled in for her 8:00 clinical practicum meeting with her supervisor, Ms. Bryce. She lingered outside Ms. Bryce's doorway, balancing a half-eaten breakfast sandwich and her cell phone while returning a text message. Ms. Bryce looked up and set aside the papers she had pulled out to work on while waiting for Abby. She waited for Abby to introduce herself, or at least explain herself, but Abby was focused on finishing off her breakfast. Eventually, Ms. Bryce introduced herself and asked Abby, who was wearing a questionably short skirt and revealing tank top, to have a seat. Abby sat down across from Ms. Bryce and began to complain about how tired she was and that it was all her roommate's fault that she was late. Ms. Bryce proceeded with the meeting, informing Abby about her expectations for the semester, as well as vital information about Abby's client. Abby appeared to be listening to what Ms. Bryce said, but she did not take a single note. What Ms. Bryce could not tell from her interaction with Abby was that she was a compassionate and intelligent student who wanted, more than anything else, to help children with autism. It was obvious that Abby was unaware about the many facets of professionalism.
>
> How could she become a successful speech-language pathologist who works in a community clinic, school system, or medical facility? If Abby did not get some instruction in professional appearance, professional demeanor, and professional communication before practicum started, her initial clinical experience would be similar to diving into a very cold pool of water. This book is designed to make the exciting journey from student to clinician more predictable and a bit less onerous for all students, especially those like Abby.

Preparing a student for the clinical practicum experience has always been a challenge. The students come to us eager about embarking on a new and rewarding profession. They have studied some of the disorders of communication in classes and observed treatment sessions performed either by master clinicians in the field or more advanced graduate students. When the time for clinical practicum arrives, they are enthusiastic and anxious about their first foray into a clinical relationship. Unfortunately, clinical work is one of those enterprises that almost all students enter with no practical experience. By our calculations, people in the speech-language pathology major have about 3 years to complete the transition from carefree undergraduate student to competent clinical professional with a master's degree.

We asked ourselves many questions in planning this text: *Would students have a better grasp of professionalism if examples were provided and it was more clearly delineated? Wouldn't it be nice if we could forewarn students about common pitfalls in the clinical practicum process, so these could be avoided? Would students operate more efficiently in off-campus placements if we spent a little time introducing the nature of those settings before the student leaves the university environment? Would clinical reports be of higher quality if we gave examples and provided suggestions for writing and a list of common errors? Would students be less anxious if we prepared them ahead of time with examples of the clinical documentation used in medical and school settings? Would students be better able to verbally interact with clients, families, other professionals, and supervisors if we provided suggestions regarding professional verbal communication?* Clearly, we felt that the answers to our questions would no doubt be in the affirmative.

This textbook was designed to help speech-language pathology students as they approach and journey through the clinical practicum experience. There are several major characteristics that distinguish our textbook. First, we wanted to provide the student with a clear understanding of professional demeanor common to speech-language pathologists. It is our view that such professionalism is largely communicated through a variety of modalities. For instance, a person's behavior, written communications, and verbal communications are perceived by others as significant indices of professionalism. Actions can include such varied components as appearance, ethical behavior, decision making, planning clinical work, and nonverbal communica-

tion skills. Actions, as they say, often speak louder than words. Written communications range from various clinical reports to progress notes and e-mails. We project our level of professionalism every time we write any type of clinical documentation. Verbal communication with clients, families, other professionals, and supervisors is the means by which we provide information, obtain information, counsel, and solve problems related to clinical activity. Because the features of professional behavior, professional writing, and professional speaking are so important in defining a professional, we elected to name this book *Professional Communication in Speech-Language Pathology: How to Write, Talk, and Act Like a Clinician.* In this third edition of the text, we have revised, updated, and expanded upon the original text to include up-to-date research and current trends in clinical practicum.

A second characteristic of this book involves the detailed information of different practicum settings. Since clinical practicum is different from any other experience these students have encountered, it is important to provide a road map of where they are headed in the process of learning to be a competent clinician. For this reason, we have chosen to discuss three practicum settings in almost every chapter: (a) university clinics, (b) medical settings, and (c) public school settings. The chapters provide examples of professional written communication that are unique to each type of workplace. Clinical documentation is similar yet different across these work settings and students should be aware of those variations before they experience an off-campus placement. But the information in this text goes beyond paperwork. We discuss professional verbal communication when interacting with clients, families, other professionals, and supervisors across work settings.

A third characteristic in almost every chapter is our delineation of proactive suggestions that are helpful to the student in navigating the various settings of clinical practicum. In this way, the book serves as a kind of survival guide to clinical practicum because we discuss common problems across settings and ways to avoid them. If we expect students to perform well across different practicum experiences, then we should tell them how their behavior and documentation should change in these settings as compared to the university clinic. In many cases, it is as simple as just listing things to do and not do. Ironically, many of the issues in practicum settings are caused by poor communication. Fortunately, it is also professional communication that plays a major role in solving practicum difficulties.

The final characteristic of this book is that we attempted to write it in a student-friendly style with copious examples and vignettes to help the student understand the material not only intellectually, but practically as well. Many books on clinical practicum are compilations of rules, references, regulations, and writing exercises that, while certainly important, are often difficult to digest. This book generally discusses most of these issues, but also illustrates them in a practical and interesting way. We hope the text can be useful as part of the smooth transition from novice student to a respected speech-language pathologist.

SECTION I

Introduction to Professional Communication, Clinical Practicum Sites, and Ethics

1

The Nature of Professionalism and Professional Communication

Introduction

The field of speech-language pathology is among the distinguished and respected helping professions. Speech-language pathologists (SLPs) work alongside a diverse group of related professionals in a variety of settings to assess and treat patients across the life span. No matter the setting, "professional" should be a term that describes us, so we need to have a clear understanding of the concept. But when we think of *professionalism*, what does this really mean? Typically, a person knows if the treatment being received is professional and can easily distinguish unprofessional behavior on the part of a service provider. However, explaining what it means to act professionally is as elusive as reaching a consensus on a common definition. We wanted to investigate what students and clinicians thought, and we included a sampling in the box below.

"Conducting oneself in a manner that brings respect to the profession and reflects well on your fellow colleagues. It's a line I have trouble with and constantly cross over."

"Professionalism is being kind and respectful when other people are being unprofessional."

"It's a behavior represented by actions of collegiality and ethical conduct."

Professionalism: "the skill, judgment, and polite behavior that is expected from a person who is trained to do a job well." Merriam-Webster's Dictionary

According to Cornett (2006, p. 1), "We demonstrate professionalism by attitudes, knowledge, and behaviors that reflect a multi-faceted approach to the standards, regulations, and principles underlying successful clinical practice." She continues that "inquiry, introspection, and integrity" are critical components of professionalism. Professionalism requires that you take the initiative to assess yourself during and following each interaction to strive to improve your skills. It is typical that some students naturally have strengths in some areas, as well as areas to improve upon.

The literature from many health-related disciplines is concerned with professionalism both at the level of training programs and in the clinical practice after graduation. For example, fields such as medicine (American Academy of Pediatrics, 2007), occupational therapy (Randolph, 2003), pharmacy (Hammer, Berger, & Beardsley, 2003), and nursing (Clooman, Davis, & Burnett, 1999) all view professionalism as a critical variable in clinical practice and in training programs. But it is not only in so-called "white collar" positions that professionalism is important. Even in jobs that are technically not "professional," we have certain standards of demeanor that are expected. For example, when you take your car in for repair you expect a certain degree of professionalism from the employees. We expect restaurant employees to behave professionally when serving customers. Professional behavior is an important part of every job from plumbing and carpentry to lawn maintenance and selling of automobiles. In all of these fields we expect the practitioners to have certain knowledge and skills that allow them to competently perform the job, and we expect to be treated with respect. If these expectations are not met, people tend to not return for additional services.

It should be no surprise to students that professionalism is an important and critical component in the practice of speech-language pathology. When clients and other professionals interact with the SLP, there are certain expectations for professionalism. What are some practical ways you can show that you are a professional? The general public expects an SLP to work in a physical setting with an appearance that instills confidence in clients and represents the professional as someone to be respected as a clinician. The language we use with clients and people from other disciplines should be professional in tone and content. The reports we generate in the course of assessment and treatment of patients should reflect the specialization and integrity of our field. Wilkinson, Wade, and Knock (2009) identified several themes when researching the definition of professionalism. These included honesty/integrity, confidentiality, respect, demeanor, empathy/rapport, organization, punctuality, and responsibility.

Professionalism is not just about how clients and other disciplines perceive us; it is also about how it makes others feel about themselves. If you treat a client with empathy and respect, it will create an environment that is conducive to positive clinical change. Conversely, a client who feels disrespected, judged, or misunderstood may have decreased motivation or participation in therapy activities.

You can see that professionalism is expected not only of seasoned clinicians, but of clinicians in training as well. One objective of this book is to help students realize the importance of professionalism in becoming an SLP and how one's behavior, language, and writing are important factors in becoming a professional. You may be wondering why someone would not choose to act professional. It may be ignorance regarding a certain area or a choice to take an easier, more convenient route.

It is not difficult to recognize unprofessional demeanor, as illustrated by this account by Joseph Berkley, a businessman who is suffering from depression.

I was seeking help for my depression, so I searched online for "professional counseling services" and found Dr. Beck. When I arrived at the office, I found the receptionist complaining on her cell phone about the patient she had just checked out. After several minutes, she got off the phone and glanced up at me. When I told her I had an appointment with Dr. Beck, she told me to follow the signs to room 112. I navigated my way through the halls, found room 112, and knocked on the door. A loud voice from inside the room yelled, "Who is it?" I felt uncomfortable announcing my name for others to hear, so I replied softly as I opened the door. Room 112 revealed a man sitting behind a cluttered desk in a t-shirt and sweatpants, finishing a bag of potato chips. Cluttering the desk were old files and paperwork from previous patients. He greeted me by saying, "What's your name, again? I didn't have time to look at my notes." It took me months to work up the courage to make an appointment with a counselor, and now I'm doubtful if this person I'm sitting across from is someone I can trust to help me. It became clear that professionalism is not conferred on a person by simply earning a degree.

The extreme example above illustrates lack of professionalism on many levels. The next day, Joseph tells us of his second attempt at finding help.

I had postponed making an appointment with a psychologist for months now. Hesitantly, I opened the double doors to Dr. Tyson's office building and walked up to the receptionist's window. The receptionist welcomed me to the office as she handed me an information packet to complete. After I signed in, she told me Dr. Tyson was expecting me and invited me to have a seat in the waiting room. Five minutes later,

before I could even crack open the book I'd brought to pass the time, a man in a freshly pressed suit emerged from behind the waiting room door. He walked directly to me and introduced himself. I put away my book and followed him out of the waiting room. Dr. Tyson escorted me to his office while we discussed our mutual appreciation for the crisp fall weather outside. We arrived at his office, a modest, yet tidy, room warmly lit by the natural light coming in through the window. Dr. Tyson asked me to have a seat and explained his goals for the session. He then asked me questions related to the concerns I had expressed over the phone. It was clear that he was sincerely interested in me as a person, not just another patient, and I felt the fear and hesitancy I had built up for so long start to disappear.

The overall difference between these two vignettes could be described in terms of physical appearances of the offices, demeanor of the office staff, the appearance of the psychologists, and the language used by the psychologists. However, an overall discriminating variable between the two scenarios is the construct of professionalism. In one situation, professional behavior was lacking, and in the other it was not. Again, we know professionalism when we see it, but it is difficult to exactly quantify. That is probably because being professional involves many variables that all interact in complex ways. There are certain characteristics of a professional that not only include duties (e.g., assessment and treatment in the case of the SLP), but also interactions (engagements) and personal attributes (character or skill).

One common thread running through the concept of professionalism is the idea that it is demonstrated largely through various forms of communication. The physical properties of a clinical environment and your appearance communicate important information about professionalism, as illustrated in the vignettes. Nonverbal communication can indicate confidence and expertise, as well as empathy for the client. Verbal communication with clients and other professionals can be a clear indication of a clinician's knowledge about the field and ability to perform assessment and treatment activities. Finally, written communication (e.g., letters, reports, treatment plans,

progress notes) represents the clinician to others when face-to-face interactions are not possible. The notion of communication is inseparable from the construct of professionalism. It is how professionalism manifests itself to clients and other professionals. Thus, it is not simply a coincidence that we have used the term *professional communication* in the title of this textbook. The term is very broad and includes both written as well as verbal interactions. Figure 1–1 shows examples of professional communi-

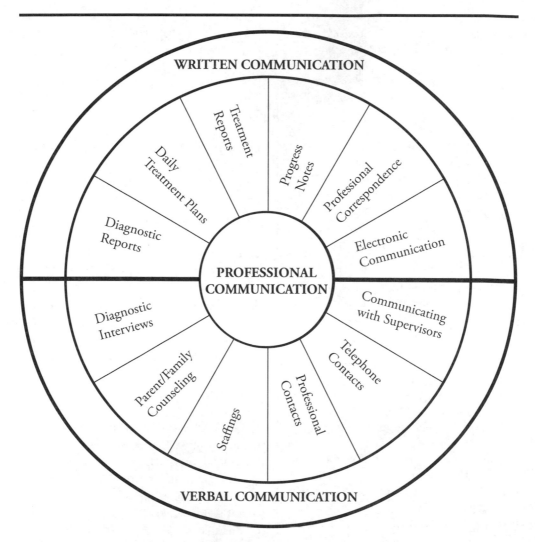

Figure 1–1. The two modalities of professional communication.

cation that represent the written and verbal modalities. Although we will be spending more time on the written forms of professional communication, it is important to address verbal communication as well. Let us spend a little time discussing the types of professional communication illustrated in Figure 1–1. In subsequent chapters of the present text we cover each of these areas in more detail.

Professional Written Communication

Both students and professionals are required to generate professional documents related to evaluations, treatment planning, and treatment reporting. All of the following reports may be shared with patients, caregivers, and allied professionals to ensure the highest quality of care. In addition, paperwork is required by third-party payers. Depending on your setting, the clinical record may be electronic or written. Figure 1–1 shows several important areas of professional written communication:

1. **Diagnostic reports:** These are clinical reports that summarize the results of a formal assessment of communication abilities, including standardized and nonstandardized testing. The diagnostic report paints a clear picture of the patient's communication abilities, including strengths and weaknesses. It becomes part of a patient's clinical record and is often transmitted, with patient permission, to other professionals. Our reports represent not only the student who wrote them, but the student's clinical supervisor and the facility (university, hospital, school system) that performed the assessment.

2. **Daily treatment plans:** Students in training are often required to develop written goals and procedures for a session in the form of a treatment plan that is submitted to the clinical supervisor for review and approval. The treatment plan outlines the plan for the therapy session with regard to goals and procedures. Students may also be asked to include rationales from theory or research for goal selection and the use of particular procedures in the treatment plan. The treatment plan should represent the result of considerable thought by the student after reviewing the case information, appropriate textbooks, class notes on the appropriate disorder, and discussions with the clinical supervisor.

3. **Treatment reports:** These reports are designed to summarize the progress of a patient in a treatment program and address changes in behavior for goals and objectives of therapy over a period of time. These reports become part of a patient's file and serve to communicate the treatment approach and progress to other professionals or future students who will provide treatment in subsequent semesters. For example, a patient being seen in the university clinic may also be seen in the public schools, and treatment reports are routinely sent to the SLP in the school system to make him or her aware of the patient's progress at the university.

4. **Progress notes:** Progress notes are short synopses written on a session by session, weekly, or monthly basis. They are part of the clinical record and summarize the patient's performance and progress toward short-term goals, benchmarks, and objectives. Progress notes are representative of the data and outcomes of therapy sessions and may be shared

with any part of the team of professionals involved in treating the client.

5. **Professional correspondence:** These are letters written to referral sources, parents, family members, or other professionals discussing general clinical matters or clinical issues related to a particular patient. Sometimes this correspondence is as simple as expressing appreciation for a referral from another professional. For instance, a physician may refer a patient with vocal nodules for voice therapy to the university clinic. It is always important to thank other professionals for referrals so that a good working relationship is maintained. You might also write a letter to a physician to whom you are referring a patient from the university clinic that explains their communication abilities. There are many different types of clinical correspondence, and it is important that each be handled in a professional manner.

6. **Electronic communication:** Electronic mail or facsimile machines are sometimes used to relate clinical information to other professionals. Although we do not typically send reports via e-mail, it is important that any correspondence with other professionals or patients be done in as professional a manner as possible. E-mail between allied professionals is prolific, and the SLP may frequently communicate short summaries of patient progress or questions regarding the patient's performance in other areas. It is not unusual for reports to be faxed between clinical settings, but as in any electronic communication, the importance of maintaining confidentiality of patient information is paramount.

In all six areas mentioned above, the SLP is expected to adhere to specific professional guidelines regarding types of language used, protection of confidential information, and format requirements. The guidelines are similar across the six forms of professional written communication, but there are also subtle differences. These guidelines are discussed in more detail in later chapters of this text.

In all settings, you should acknowledge that the clinical record is a communication tool that is shared among a group of professionals, all of whom serve the patient. This team of allied professionals includes teachers, therapists, physicians, psychologists, and other medical professionals. It always includes the patient and the patient's family or caregivers. The record, which includes your reports, is a representation of the quality of service you provide and is vital for others to reference when determining what is best for the client. Paul (1994) cites the following as purposes of documentation:

- Support diagnosis and treatment (including medical necessity and need for skilled services)
- Describe client progress
- Justify discharge from treatment
- Support reimbursement
- Communicate with other professionals
- Justify clinical decisions
- Protect legal interests of client, service provider, and facility
- Serve as evidence in a court of law
- Provide data for research (i.e., efficacy)

You might be asking yourself, "How difficult can it be to learn how to write all these different kinds of documents?" You may have been an excellent student in English composition but, unfortunately, clinical writing is quite different from generating a term paper or short story. In professional writing you will be expected to use professional terminology, write the document in the appropriate format, and employ specific descriptions of a patient's performance in reporting assessment or treatment results. You might be saying, "Why can't I just write it my way instead of using all these technical terms and strange formats?" Failure to understand the importance of clinical writing as a unique genre has not only led to poor grades in clinical practicum, but ultimately a difficult transition to your first job. It is important for you to realize early on that clinical supervisors and future employers take professional written communication very seriously. Professional writing or reporting is always included on clinical practicum grading forms, and students are evaluated on the punctuality of submitting paperwork, the quality of their professional writing, the completeness of the reports, and the appropriateness of the paperwork for the work setting. Ironically, although students are certain to be evaluated on these important facets of clinical ability, there is often little direct classroom teaching that focuses on professional writing. Textbooks most often devote a single chapter or part of a chapter to professional writing, and this is typically not enough exposure to prepare students for different types of reports (e.g., evaluation, treatment) or paperwork peculiar to a specific work setting (e.g., Individualized Education Program [IEP]/ Individualized Family Service Plan [IFSP] in schools, plans of care in medical settings, etc.). Seeking examples of documentation and specific feedback from supervisors and peers is crucial to being a competent clinical writer.

Students have said that report writing style varies considerably by supervisor, and that what might be perfectly acceptable for one person may not be acceptable for another. An additional difficulty occurs when the student leaves the insulated setting of the university clinic for off-campus practicum. The student will soon learn that in the "real world," evaluation, treatment, and report writing are quite different from what goes on at the university. As such, students are buffeted about from one supervisor to another and one setting to another, and finally they "learn" professional writing through a process that involves much trial and error and some bruising of their egos. The present authors feel that professional writing is somewhat of a mystery to beginning students. We find it paradoxical that students are expected to learn professional writing largely through trial and error and with precious few resources that adequately address professional writing issues. This is precisely why we feel that a more proactive approach needs to be taken to professional writing in the form of a guidebook that is specifically directed to students in training. It is our hope that such a resource will demystify professional writing, illustrate appropriate formats used across work settings, discuss common errors that students tend to make, and show students examples of all the types of paperwork they will encounter at the levels of their training. It is not possible to totally eliminate the frustrations associated with report writing for both students and supervisors because there is a certain amount of trial and error that *must* be experienced to learn this elusive craft. It is not necessary, however, to leave the entire process to chance. If we can provide explicit information in terms of report formats, typical writing errors, and professional language, the student can be more proactive and produce an initial effort that is closer to the desired target.

Professional Verbal Communication

The bottom portion of Figure 1–1 illustrates that professional communication is not confined to the written modality. There are many occasions on which students are expected to communicate verbally with parents, family members, or other professionals both in person and over the telephone. You might be thinking, "I already know how to talk to people. What is different about talking to people in a clinical setting?" Again, there is a certain professional demeanor and use of language that is expected in a clinical setting. There are certain terms to use, just as in clinical reports. There is even a "format" for what to talk about in certain situations.

Being professional is sometimes associated with a high level of formality; however, this is not always the case. Of course, interactions should begin formally, but after rapport is built and a trusting relationship has been established, the formality of your interaction style may shift. Some individuals may find it incredibly daunting to be in the hospital or clinic and may require you to be more informal to put them at ease. Others may find reassurance in formal interactions as evidence of your competence as a clinician. As the student and clinician, it is your responsibility to take the lead from your supervisors and patients. We briefly mention the areas of verbal professional communication below:

1. **Diagnostic interviews:** No matter what type of patient you see in a diagnostic evaluation, the interaction always begins with an interview. In some cases, it may occur over the phone, as well as in person. In the context of the diagnostic interview you will be interested in directing the conversation so that you can obtain information, give information, and explain the assessment results to the client/family (Pindzola, Plexico, & Haynes, 2016). These interviews require organization, planning, and skill that few people innately possess, and prowess comes with practice. Later in the text we talk more about professional communication in diagnostic interviews. For now, however, it is enough to realize that professional communication involves talking as well as writing.

2. **Patient/caregiver counseling:** There are many occasions when we talk to patients and family members or caregivers about diagnoses, treatment progress, referrals, or enlisting their help with the therapy program. This can be a very sensitive area to broach since it involves discussion of patient abilities and a wealth of information that is likely unfamiliar to those we are speaking to. For that reason, great care must be taken to communicate clearly and with respect.

3. **Staffings:** In many work settings, a variety of professionals from different disciplines gather together to discuss a particular client. This may also be called a team meeting or grand rounds discussion. For example, it would not be unusual to see a staffing that included an SLP, psychologist, classroom teacher, parent, and occupational therapist. In medical settings, the staffing can include various therapists, the physician, nurse, case manager, and dietician. Each professional contributes unique information to the staffing and is expected to communicate professionally. There are guidelines for professional communication in such settings, and we discuss these in later sections.

4. **Professional contacts:** Often, the SLP will be asked to talk with physicians, physical therapists, radiologists, psychologists, teachers, audiologists, special educators, and other professionals. These discussions may involve you summarizing your assessment or treatment of a client or making an appropriate referral. This is frequently accomplished over the phone but can also take place in person.

5. **Communicating with supervisors:** As a student, you will have many opportunities to communicate with clinical supervisors, special education coordinators, directors of SLP in medical settings, principals of schools, and other people to whom you have to answer for your activities. Professional verbal communication is important in all of these situations and helps you make a good first impression. You may be explaining the progress of a particular

case or lobbying for monetary support to purchase tests and materials. Professional verbal communication is a key ingredient to establishing yourself as a competent and respectable student and employee.

Shared Components of Professional Written and Verbal Communication

Figure 1–2 shows some shared components of professional written and verbal communication. By shared components, we mean that certain commonalities exist between the written and verbal expressions of professional communication. In many ways, these components help to differentiate a conversation with a personal friend, rather than one with a patient. We briefly discuss each below:

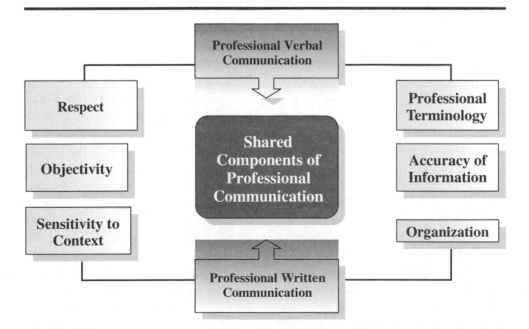

Figure 1–2. Shared components of professional written and verbal communication.

1. **Professional terminology:** In both verbal and written professional communication, it is expected that appropriate terminology will be used by the SLP. We use terms such as *oral cavity* instead of *mouth* or *phonemes* instead of *sounds*. The SLP will discuss syntax, semantics, pragmatics, and morphology when talking about language. In both verbal and written interactions, professional terms are appropriate to use, depending on the audience. As we discuss later, the context of communication in terms of where you are talking and to whom you are talking is important to consider when using discipline-specific terminology.

2. **Accuracy of information:** It is assumed that any professional communication will contain accurate information, whether it is a verbal interaction or a clinical report. If a professional is asked how a child scored on a test, it would not be appropriate to say, "I think he scored in the 5th percentile, or maybe the 40th." If you can't remember the score, do not speculate but consult the report. You should never hesitate to reference data or test results when you are not confident in what you are reporting. In a written report, we describe assessment and treatment information accurately using test scores and descriptions of behavior because we do not want to say something without reliable and valid evidence. Professionals always double-check the scoring and reporting of test data to ensure that they are accurate. There is typically a portion of a clinical report that allows a practitioner an opportunity to discuss "clinical impressions." This section of a report, however, is clearly demarcated from the parts of the writing that describe test scores and more objective information. Professional communication is highly concerned with accuracy.

3. **Organization:** Professional communication should be orderly both in the written and verbal modalities. If you are part of a multidisciplinary staffing and are asked to talk about a child's language disorder and progress in treatment, the other professionals present do not expect you to embark on an unorganized stream of consciousness rant about the client. They expect you to provide some background information, talk a bit about assessment, outline the treatment goals, and discuss progress in therapy. Even though you are talking, there is a basic organization that is expected from a professional. Obviously, in clinical reports, there is a format that is unique to the work setting that guides your writing. Again, it is not like writing a casual note to a friend but a highly organized summary of specific information written in professional language.

4. **Respect:** One of the hallmarks of professional communication involves showing respect for the patient, family, or other professional. This is not merely a courtesy but is demanded by the codes of ethics of virtually every professional organization. This is why we usually refer to adult clients as "Mr. Smith" or "Mrs. Jones" rather than "Charlie" or "Edith." Certainly, as a clinical relationship develops, we may refer to patients by their first names, but only when it is mutually agreeable and appropriate. Respect is also shown when we take into account the feelings and attitudes of others in the course of our interactions. We want to build trust, not offend patients or other professionals with either our reports or verbal interactions. We show respect when we listen to the opinions of other professionals about our patients and when we listen to our patients as they tell us about

their concerns. Very often, patients and caregivers feel vulnerable as they share details regarding their personal lives or medical histories. It is vital that we pay attention to our nonverbal behavior to ensure we are not projecting a sense of judgment or disapproval. In Chapter 12, we address interaction styles as they relate to patients of diverse cultural backgrounds. Respect is also shown in the quality of our physical facilities, the comfort of the chairs, and the reading material provided in our waiting rooms. After all, making patients wait in the squalor of a filthy, disorganized waiting room is a sign of disrespect to our clients. If we show up late for a therapy appointment and our materials are disorganized, we are saying to our patients that we do not think enough of them to take the time to prepare for their sessions.

5. **Objectivity:** Part of professional communication, whether verbal or in writing, is that it is unbiased and reflects objective facts as much as possible. We assume that the professional SLP will gather appropriate information in an assessment and objectively interpret the data. Professional communication is not as much about a clinician's opinion as it is about evidence that can be documented. Professionals should never say something for which there is not adequate evidence or misrepresent the information that they are communicating. For instance, a clinician should not state that a child has cognitive limitations or autism without the appropriate diagnosis. For instance, if we said, "Edward has behavior problems," it could be construed by the reader that he had actually been diagnosed with behavior disorder. It is much better to describe any behaviors that are of concern rather than provide an inaccurate

supposition. In this case, you could note "Edward attempted to hit the clinician when she presented stimuli during testing." You should certainly make a referral to another professional if you feel that a patient is displaying characteristics of a disorder that is outside your scope of practice to diagnose.

6. **Sensitivity to context:** Contextual sensitivity affects professional communication in several ways. First, it is important to communicate in an appropriate way based on the setting in which the communication takes place. For example, in verbal communication in a hospital setting, certain words are used that are unique to that environment. One can use abbreviations such as *NICU*, *FIM scores*, *ADL*, *p.r.n.*, and *ROM*, and people in the medical setting will know what you are talking about. However, if you use these terms in the public school setting, teachers might not know what you mean. Conversely, in the school system you might use terms such as *Title I*, *Bloom's taxonomy*, *RTI*, *IEP*, and *IDEA*, which would be less understood in medical settings. At any rate, sensitivity to the context is an important influence on professional verbal communication. Context also has a large effect on professional written communication. For instance, the format for written reports and progress notes differs dramatically among university clinics, medical settings, and school environments. Your written communication must change depending on the context of the work setting. A second implication of sensitivity to context in professional communication concerns the person to whom you are talking or writing. For example, parents and caregivers are a very diverse group in terms of social status and educational level. You cannot explain the results of

an evaluation the same way to a person with a graduate degree and another person with an eighth grade education, yet you have to do it professionally in both cases. A key to figuring out how to share information is to listen. Listening to the ways patients or caregivers explain the communication problem and the questions they ask will give you valuable insight regarding how to educate them. In written communication, reports tend to be written in professional language and would not be understandable by some parents. In these cases, a "parent-friendly" summary letter may be sent or a follow-up phone call may be made to explain the critical information in the report. When talking to other professionals, we must discriminate which terminology people from other disciplines may and may not understand and adjust our conversation appropriately. If we are sharing results from an evaluation, an explanation about terms specific to our discipline might be necessary to allow someone from occupational therapy to benefit from the information shared. Thus, professional verbal and written communication must change with the context in which we are communicating, both in terms of the setting and the person to whom we are talking.

How do students learn about professional verbal communication? This is an interesting question because there are typically no specific courses that address the issue. Most students learn how to communicate professionally by modeling clinical supervisors and watching students who are further along in their training. Watching the behavior of an experienced clinician who is communicating professionally goes a long way toward teaching less experienced students how to act in a clinical role. In most cases, beginning students are not given the responsibility to independently interview patients, meet with other professionals, or counsel families. Students usually start by observing such activities during their required hours of observation. When students receive their first clinical assignments, they typically are asked to conduct certain parts of interviews, staffing presentations, or counseling efforts while being guided by their supervisor. A student progressing through the training program is given a greater role in professional verbal communication, and any missteps are pointed out after the interaction by the clinical supervisor. A good strategy for any student in training is to take advantage of every opportunity to observe your clinical faculty engaged in professional communication with patients, families, or allied professionals. You will most likely see positive and negative examples, both of which will help you refine your own level of professionalism.

In the upcoming chapters we discuss both written and verbal communication in more detail to provide some general guidelines that will help you navigate your training program. As you will see in the next chapter, there is no one way to write reports, nor is there just one format for verbal interaction.

2

Learning as They Change the Rules: The Many Faces of Clinical Practicum

University Supervisor: "You must dress professionally when you are working with clients."

Hospital Supervisor: "You can wear scrubs to work."

University Supervisor: "Your report was not long enough and did not have sufficient detail."

Hospital Supervisor: "Your report was far too long."

University Practicum Student: "My client has been coming to the clinic for 5 years."

Hospital Practicum Student: "We see our patients in acute care for only a few days."

University Supervisor: "Always take a detailed case history and put it in your report."

Hospital Supervisor: "Our patients usually can't give a reliable case history. All we have is a couple of lines in the chart written by the case worker."

University Supervisor: "Administer standardized tests in their entirety according to the instruction manual so you can compare the scores to norms."

Hospital Supervisor: "We rarely give a complete standardized test. We have taken tasks from many tests and made up our own assessment protocol."

University Practicum Student: "I spent 3 hours last night developing a home program for my client."

Skilled Nursing Practicum Student: "Most of my patients will never go home, so they don't need a home program."

University Practicum Student: "My client's spouse wants to talk after each session to learn how she can better help him find his words and improve his speech."

School Practicum Student: "We rarely see parents, except at IEP meetings once a year."

University Practicum Student: "My last diagnostic report was eight pages long."

Rehabilitation Practicum Student: "For my last report, I clicked boxes on a one-page form."

University Practicum Student: "I see this little boy individually and it's hard to develop enough activities for an hour session to keep him busy."

School Practicum Student: "I work mostly with kids in groups for less than half an hour."

University Practicum Student: "I have five goals I'm working on with my client that are based on testing and parent concerns."

School Practicum Student: "My goals have to be educationally relevant and related to federally mandated benchmarks."

University Practicum Student: "I'm working with a kid who substitutes w/r."

School Practicum Student: "In my school, kids with /r/ problems don't qualify for services."

University Practicum Student: "The client I work with brought me the sweetest thank-you note and my favorite cookies for working with him this semester."

Skilled Nursing Practicum Student: "Most of my patients have cognitive deficits and don't remember my name."

Introduction

The title of this chapter suggests that students in communication sciences and disorders will be confronted with many changes. On the surface, the statements from students and supervisors in the above box might seem in diametrical opposition. How can a clinical practice be acceptable to one student or supervisor on one occasion and unacceptable on another? Why is there such diversity in everything including clients, administrative procedures, opinions of supervisors, paperwork requirements, and types of therapy? The different perspectives illustrated above would seem to be a recipe for cognitive dissonance in our practicum students. Is it all part of an insidious plot to drive you completely insane? How can you be successful if the rules keep changing? Do not despair. We are here to help you.

If you are reading this book as part of your curriculum in communication sciences and disorders, we would like to welcome you to an exciting, diverse, and challenging profession. Over many years of teaching in a university training program, we have seen scores of students who decided to major in speech-language pathology. We have watched with great interest as they passed through the various phases of the curriculum and emerged on the other end as competent professionals. Through their training we saw the wonder on their faces as they began to understand the marvelous process of communication, as well as the life-altering impact the disorders can have on a person's quality of life. We watched their first tentative therapy sessions and then saw them return from their internship showing all the confidence of a seasoned veteran. Over the course of training, however, we also were witness to many looks of consternation, confusion, and frustra-

tion as these students approached specific transition points in their programs. Much of their disquiet revolved more around the practicum experience than the coursework. Classes, after so long, become easy to deal with, and students accepted into graduate programs usually have well-developed strategies for classroom success. Clinical practice, however, is a different matter. Here you are, after all those courses, actually working with someone for the first time. Let us assure you that everyone in this situation is uncertain, apprehensive, excited, and clueless. One of the things that make practicum so uncertain is that there is no one way to do it. If there were a magic formula for planning, executing, and reporting every disorder the same way, it would certainly be easier. But there are different types of clients, multiple disorders, varied supervisors, and diverse practicum settings, all of which make clinical work confusing to the novice therapist. Students have reported several specific sources of frustration with their practicum experiences over the years. First, they do not seem to understand how the university training program interfaces with other settings to form the overall practicum experience. Students do not seem to appreciate the "big picture" of why the university training program teaches certain things and why other settings may conduct business quite differently.

A second problem for students is making the adjustment between practicum settings as they go through clinical training. Each setting has a different type of caseload, physical characteristics, professionals, and requirements for clinical reporting. The student is exposed to long narrative reports in the university clinic, chart notes in medical settings, and Individualized Education Programs (IEPs) in school systems. Just when you reach a certain degree of comfort in one format, you are asked to provide therapy and complete clinical reporting in a totally different way. It is not that we are trying to drive you completely mad; there are logical reasons for these inconsistencies. Any accredited program in communication disorders must ensure that you obtain practicum experiences across different types of clinical environments. Thus, it should not be a surprise that you will transition from the comfortable venue of the university speech and hearing clinic and be transplanted into a rehabilitation hospital in the space of just a semester. Virtually everything is different, and even though you knew on some level that practicum sites would differ, you had no way to prepare yourself for such a startling transition. Our motivation behind writing this book was to help ease some of the transitions for students who are moved abruptly across different practicum settings. One of the most frustrating aspects of the changing terrain is the different paperwork requirements and professional behaviors that are required. We thought that if students could get a preview of the requirements across sites, the transitions would be a bit easier. That is why we have organized this book to some degree by work setting. So, if you are headed to a hospital next semester, check out the parts of the book that deal with reporting and behavior in medical settings. If you are assigned to a local elementary school, look at the sections devoted to educational settings. One thing is certain: each setting has its own unique culture and set of requirements for behavior and paperwork. Granted, you will not fully understand the nature of these things until you have spent a couple of weeks in a new practicum setting, but knowing a bit about what to expect will lessen your frustration and apprehension. This book is primarily concerned with professional communication across work settings, but

we also provide some suggestions on how to survive as a practicum student in each workplace.

In the United States, there are approximately 300 training programs in speech-language pathology (SLP) that are accredited by the American Speech-Language-Hearing Association (ASHA). Within the context of each of these programs, undergraduate and graduate level students must earn a minimum of 400 hours of supervised clinical practicum across at least three different clinical settings. This means that the student must gain experience in university clinics, hospitals, community clinics, schools, skilled nursing facilities, or rehabilitation facilities with a wide diversity of clients representing many different types of communication disorders. Across all of these practicum settings and types of clients, the student in training is expected to participate in a variety of professional communications, both verbal and written.

Clinical Settings

As stated earlier, students are expected to participate in practicum experiences across a variety of work settings before they earn their graduate degree. The three most common types of clinical environments that students will encounter are university clinics, medical settings (e.g., hospitals, rehabilitation centers, nursing homes), and public schools. When students are initially placed in each of these three types of settings, they instantly notice that there are significant differences among the environments in terms of clients, the pace of assessment/ treatment, and paperwork requirements. We would like to take some time now to clarify a couple of misconceptions students often have about how these settings relate to one another. First, it is important to realize that each setting is unique, and there is no way that a particular type of facility can substitute for a different type of operation. For example, the university setting is typically a community clinic and cannot operate as a school or hospital. There is no way we can place beds in a university clinic or do instrumental studies of swallowing. Likewise, we cannot use the university to act as an elementary school for large groups of children with communication disorders. University clinic training acts as a sheltered environment for initial clinical experiences and is not meant to substitute for or emulate medical or educational placements. In fact, some training programs do not even have an on-campus clinic and students will have to get all of their training off-site.

As mentioned above, students are sent to off-campus sites to gain unique clinical experiences that are not available in a university clinic. Sometimes students will be concerned that they have not been given practicum experience with swallowing disorders at the university clinic and have engaged only in classroom study of the issues. When they go to a hospital, they have their first hands-on experience with dysphagia. Of course, that is exactly why they were sent to the medical placement: to obtain experience that is not available in the university clinic. Another misconception is that no one type of setting is superior to another. The sites are merely different. Students sometimes come back to the university after an off-campus medical placement and tell us that the experiences they had in the training program do not reflect the "real world" of the hospital or rehabilitation center. Of course, these medical placements do not reflect the real world of the public schools either, and vice versa. Students

often forget that the university training program has a goal of exposing them to the real world, and this is accomplished through off-campus placements and internship experiences. Thus, it is simply not accurate to say that the university does not reflect real-world practices; it systematically provides students with exposure to other settings through practicum experiences. University training programs are neither better nor worse than other placements; they are just different. At the university we try to present all of the relevant information and we may not necessarily tailor it to a particular work setting. That part is done by the supervising professionals who are working in medical settings and school systems. There may be many scientifically supported approaches to assessment and treatment that are "ideal," and these may have to be modified to be appropriate in medical or school settings. Thus, students should not think of one setting as being wrong when there are simply different ways of approaching clinical work in each one.

Some of the differences among settings flow from regulatory agencies (e.g., ASHA, Medicare, private insurance, Department of Education, etc.), and others stem from the "culture" of each work environment. Table 2–1 shows the differences in regulatory agencies that dictate how each setting operates. University training programs are run a particular way because ASHA accreditation hangs in the balance. Medical settings are hamstrung by federal and state regulations, Medicare/Medicaid regulations, and insurance companies. Educational settings have a myriad of federal and state regulations to abide by in conducting their business. Table 2–2 depicts some of the differences in clinical operation in terms of caseload, supervision, and reporting. Just considering these primal differences among

Table 2–1. Practicum Setting Comparison Chart: Regulatory Control

	University	Medical	School
ASHA Regulations	• Heavily regulated by ASHA • Must train knowledge and skills • Accreditation requirements • Professional practice standards	• Not regulated by ASHA • Only professional practice standards and code of ethics apply	• Not regulated by ASHA
Federal Medicare Regulations	• No Medicare regulations unless clinic is a Medicare provider	• Heavily regulated by Medicare for adult clients	• Not regulated by Medicare
Federal Medicaid Regulations	• No Medicaid regulations unless clinic is a Medicaid provider	• Heavily regulated by Medicaid for child clients	• Not all systems regulated by Medicaid unless they bill Medicaid
Federal Education Regulations	• No federal education regulations	• No federal education regulations	• Heavily regulated by federal education department
State Education Regulations	• No state education regulations	• No state education regulations	• Heavily regulated by state education department
Federal Hospital Regulations	• No federal hospital regulations	• Heavily regulated by national guidelines	• No federal hospital regulations
State Hospital Regulations	• No state hospital regulations	• Heavily regulated by state guidelines	• No state hospital regulations
Third-Party Payer Influence (e.g., insurance companies)	• Some clients use third-party payers • Some insurance carriers limit the amount and type of assessment/ treatment paid for	• Insurance companies regulate number and length of sessions paid for • Insurance companies regulate types of treatment reimbursed • Assessment and treatment are often driven by administrative regulations for billable hours	• No third-party payers

Table 2–2. Practicum Setting Comparison Chart: Clinical Operation

	University	*Medical*	*School*
Caseload Issues	• Total control of caseload • Caseload determined by number of students and faculty and availability of clinical facilities	• Typically large caseloads • Little control of caseload	• Typically large caseloads • Little control of caseload • Legal mandates to provide free services to all qualified children
Pressure to Earn Income for Clinic	• Clinic income not usually the basis for faculty salaries • Often have sliding fee scale where patients pay according to income level and family size	• Pressure to generate billable hours • Income may be used to pay salaries and benefits	• Treatment does not produce income because it is free
Time Limitations on Clinical Work	• No time limitations on length of evaluations or treatment sessions	• Limitation on amount of time that can be billed to Medicare or third-party payers	• Limitation on assessment and treatment time imposed by large caseloads and local regulations
Reports and Paperwork	• Reports are typically designed to teach clinicians to provide complete, accurate information • Reports may be lengthy with room for narrative explanations of case history information and interpretation • Greatest opportunity for lengthy reports	• Reports are extremely brief and may be limited to checklists with few opportunities for narrative • Reports may be in electronic format in a paperless environment • Least opportunity for lengthy reports	• Reports may include narratives, test scores, or, depending on the school system, a form with check boxes • Treatment reports are often the IEP • Moderate opportunity for lengthy reports

work settings should help you to understand why your practicum experiences will change dramatically depending on where you are assigned. We elaborate on each work setting in the following sections. However, we include some general suggestions for interacting with supervisors across all settings.

1. **Look the part:** When you meet with your clinical practicum supervisor for the first time, make sure that you try to appear professional. You must remember that in many cases, your practicum supervisor may have never met you before, and if there was a prior meeting, it was probably in a classroom setting. In some instances, you may never have even had a conversation with one another. So it does not hurt to dress for success and come to your first meeting with a notebook in which to jot down important information. Remember that professionalism is communicated by your appearance, your demeanor, and the language you use.

2. **Be punctual:** When you have your first meeting and meetings thereafter, make certain that you are on time. It is extremely important once you begin clinical practicum to make sure you are punctual for your scheduled cases; being on time indicates respect for your client. Your promptness for a supervisory conference may be seen as a bellwether of your clinical responsibility to clients.

3. **Be prepared by reviewing your case:** When you go for your first supervisory conference, you no doubt will have been assigned a client with whom you will be working. It is always good form to have *extensively* studied the client's file from beginning to end. Do not just read the last report and omit the historical perspective. Supervisors will often ask beginning students to summarize the case as a way of beginning the first conference. If you are not prepared, you run the risk of being perceived as uninterested and unprofessional. Even if you are not asked to summarize the case, it is good policy to be as familiar with your client as possible. Knowing your client's medical and treatment history is paramount so you can make competent decisions regarding future sessions. Usually, students tend to use the recommendations that were made in the most recent report as a template for planning their current approach to treatment. Although this is very logical, there is nothing wrong with having questions about the treatment approach that was recommended. If you find inconsistencies in the report, it is good to ask for clarification from the supervisor as to why they exist. You can make suggestions about applying concepts from your academic work to the case as well. At the very least, you should ask questions about how a procedure was actually done in treatment sessions. It is almost impossible to recreate treatment tasks in a clinical report in sufficient detail to be replicated by a new clinician. So asking your supervisor, "Can you give me an example of how this task was actually done in a session?" is not inappropriate. If you can communicate that you are prepared for your first conference, your supervisor will tend to perceive you as having a high degree of professionalism.

4. **Be prepared by reviewing class notes:** Because you reviewed the client's file, you will know the kind of disorder the client exhibits. For instance, if you are assigned a child with a language disorder, you would be wise to review your notes from the courses you took in language acquisition and language disorders. If the client has specific symptoms or is in a particular stage of language development, you should especially refresh your memory regarding course information on this stage. Your supervisor might ask you a question such as, "What is the next thing to develop

in a typically developing child at this stage of language acquisition?" It does nothing for your professional image if you shrug your shoulders and say, "I don't know." After all, you have taken several courses covering the disorders, and your inability to answer the question means that (a) you learned nothing from the course or (b) you did not prepare for the supervisory conference. Either of those reasons suggests a less than professional attitude.

5. **Be prepared to write things down:** It is important that you show that you are taking responsibility for your client and ownership of the treatment plan. A good way to communicate this to your supervisor is to take notes. We have had some students have a meeting with us to discuss therapy activities only to hurriedly ask us before their session, "What did you say again?" This not only wastes your supervisor's time but results in you not being prepared and perhaps a less than ideal treatment session. It is good practice to avoid this scenario by writing down specifics when you discuss them with your supervisor. Do not take it for granted that you will remember or falsely assume that your supervisor thinks you should not need to take notes. After you have taken the time to be prepared with thoughtful questions regarding treatment history, you should write down the answers so you will have them to go over later. You may be worried that it takes extra time to write the information down; however, we can assure you that it shows your supervisor you are prepared and conscientious. It also provides a valuable resource for you to review when planning for treatment sessions.

6. **Talk with other students or professionals if possible:** If your client is in

the university clinic and was seen previously by a student who is still around, it is valuable to contact that clinician and chat about the case. If you are in a school or medical setting, it is equally beneficial to solicit advice from professionals who are familiar with the case. You can gain much insight about the client, the treatment activities, the family, behavioral issues, room arrangement, and other information from a previous clinician. Get as much information as possible about your client, from any sources available to you, while maintaining confidentiality.

7. **Use professional language:** As much as possible, try to use appropriate terminology when talking to your supervisor. For example, do not call phonemes "speech sounds" when you know the appropriate term.

8. **Define your responsibilities:** During the first conference make certain that you know what you are expected to do each week and throughout the practicum. It goes without saying that you will be expected to be present for your therapy sessions. There are other meetings and responsibilities, however, that may not be as clear to you initially. For instance, you will probably have to schedule a supervisory conference on a weekly basis to discuss your case and your developing clinical skills. If the meeting time is ongoing from week to week, block it out on your calendar. Make sure you know what is to be done during these conferences. For example, the supervisor may want you to bring treatment data on the client's goals to each meeting. If you do not bring the data, there is little to talk about in the meeting and you are perceived as not meeting one of your professional obligations. Do you have to write progress

notes each week? Where are they, and what is the format? Are you expected to transcribe language samples periodically to monitor progress? Is there a progress report due on a particular date? When does treatment end, and when is the final report due to the supervisor? What is your role in contacting other professionals working with your case (e.g., school system, psychologist) to coordinate programs or check on generalization? What is expected of you regarding parent counseling or devising a home program to assist in generalization? All of these questions are important for you to ask or clarify if they are not already addressed by your clinical supervisor. They show that you are interested in the client and professional in your involvement. As clinical supervisors, we can tell you that we welcome as many questions as it takes for you to completely understand your responsibilities.

9. **Determine how you will be evaluated:** The interaction between you and your clinical supervisor has two major goals. First, both you and your supervisor want the client to be given appropriate services and make progress as a result. A second goal that is unique to training programs is that the supervisor wants to see your own clinical behavior change over time. It is important that you ask how and when you will be evaluated and how your grade in clinical practicum will be determined. In most cases, there are evaluation forms that your supervisor will share with you that show the behaviors and attributes she uses in grading your clinical competence. Sometimes supervisors e-mail or leave notes after sessions to provide feedback to students. Some programs evaluate students midway through the semester and again at the end. However your supervisor provides written or verbal feedback, it is critical that you get it often and early enough in the semester to make changes in your behavior. If you are not getting enough feedback, do not be shy about asking for it.

10. **Other expectations:** Be certain to clarify any expectations that go beyond the therapy session itself. For example, be familiar with clinic guidelines about infection control, disinfecting toys/materials, checking out of materials/tests, and returning the treatment room to its original condition for the next clinician. Also make sure you are aware of periodic meetings or staffings that you are expected to attend. Facilities may have specific policies and procedures that you must adhere to, and you should request clarification if needed.

The University Setting

Figure 2–1 shows a university setting, depicted as a series of "ivory towers" surrounded by several pictures. We have the ubiquitous professor lecturing to a class and another picture of a classroom using multimedia. Another picture shows a student dragging himself to the classroom with questionable motivation. The picture of the hand helping the person up the stairway symbolizes the sheltered environment of the training program where academic and clinical faculty are there to assist you if you have difficulty. Books, of course, are part of the deal in a training program, and we are aware that your tendency will be to sell them, but try to resist it so you will not have to buy them all back for your professional library. Graduation and receiving your diploma are obviously the main goals; you want to be a certified speech-language

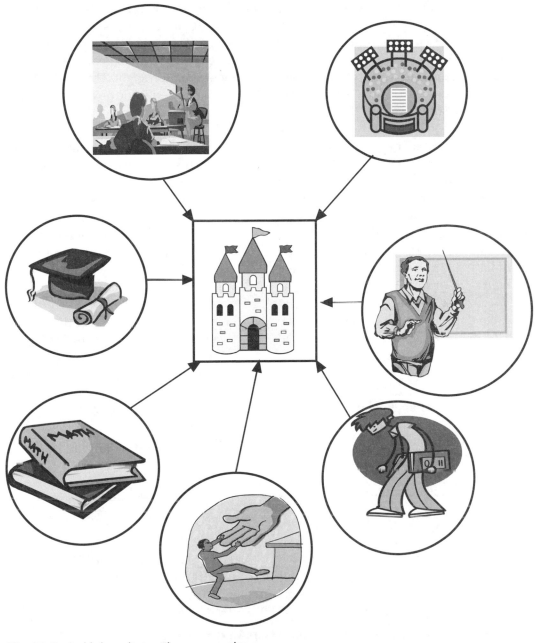

Figure 2–1. University settings are unique.

pathologist who graduated with a master's degree from an accredited program. Finally, the stadium represents some of the extracurricular activities that are part of college life. Enjoy your experience as a student, because as you reach the end of your training program, it begins to approximate the feeling of a "real job." In our program, for example, students finish their master's training with a semester-long internship in some sort of medical or educational facility where they are working full-time every day. They usually comment that they are tired at the end of the day but are thankful they do not have to study and take examinations. These same students will graduate, do their clinical fellowship (CF), and then they will no longer be students at all, but professionals with jobs, mortgages, and car payments. And take our word for it, you will long for those days when you were a student with less responsibility and much more free time. It's all part of growing up. The pictures we selected in Figure 2–1 are certainly not representative of all the experiences you might have had at the university; they were selected to portray the climate of your time in college. You will see when we begin to discuss other practicum settings that the orbit of pictures circling the hospital and school building are quite different indeed. This is because each setting has its own culture, atmosphere, and mood.

University training programs are largely designed to produce competent clinicians who are eligible for certification. Much of what goes on in the university training program is dictated by ASHA regulations and accreditation requirements. Figure 2–2 illustrates the flow of experiences in a university training program. The following are just some of the specific objectives of a university training program:

- Teach a specific knowledge base in normal processes of communication (speech science, anatomy, physiology, phonetics, language acquisition).
- Teach a specific knowledge base in disorders of communication involving phonology, language, voice, fluency, and swallowing. This knowledge base must transcend specific settings and represent the most current information and ideal standards of practice with particular disorders.
- Provide a scientific basis or rationale for assessment and treatment of communication disorders.
- Provide a sheltered environment for initial forays into clinical practice.

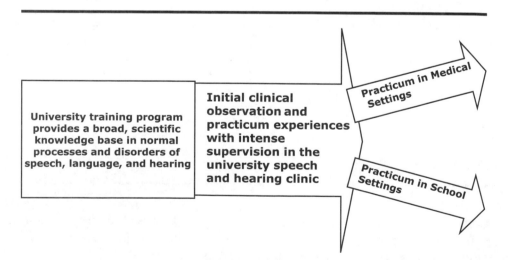

Figure 2–2. Progression of clinical training involving three settings.

- Provide students constructive feedback on developing clinical skills.
- Coordinate additional practicum experiences in unique settings for experiences that are not available in the university speech and hearing clinic.

University clinics typically have limited caseloads due to the regulations on supervision of students in training. Students must be supervised by a certified professional at least 25% of the time for treatment and 50% of the time for assessment. These requirements make it difficult for a university clinic to amass several hundred clients, due to the limitations of student clinicians and the constraint of having enough clinical supervisors. As a result, the caseloads in university clinics are small enough that clients can be offered assessment and treatment sessions that are longer than in other settings. For instance, longer diagnostic sessions are typical in the university setting because the gold standard evaluation is attempted. The students are given the opportunity to administer a variety of assessments with less time constraints than in other settings. This allows the students to develop and demonstrate the knowledge and skills required for certification by ASHA. Students and supervisors schedule time on a weekly basis to talk about the client's progress, the clinician's developing skills, and insights from class. Often a lengthier assessment results in a clearer picture of the client's strengths and needs. This is a luxury unique to the university setting, in that other settings may have large caseloads or productivity demands.

It is unique in the university setting that you will typically have little face-to-face communication with teachers, physicians, and other therapists who are also involved in the care of your client. In the public school or medical setting, it is not uncommon to spend a significant part of your day corresponding with other professionals involved in the care of your client as they are on site. Therefore, when treating clients at the university clinic, it will take some effort on your part to find an effective way of communicating with your client's teacher or other therapists to be on the same page.

A limitation of the university clinic is that this environment cannot recreate the atmosphere of a hospital or school system. It is difficult to prepare students in university clinics to handle situations involving children being pulled from classrooms or adult patients who are nonambulatory and must be transported by wheelchair to therapy. With regard to report writing, most universities take the view that students in training should produce reports with the most complete data and comprehensive narrative sections to illustrate the most that can be done with professional writing. At some point in your career, you may be asked to produce a formal report that will be used in a legal case or to establish eligibility for specific services on behalf of a client. In these cases, a simple checklist would not be the most appropriate type of report. There may be a need for explanation of the rationale for treatment and elucidation of how and why treatment targets have changed over time. Thus, university clinics are relatively sheltered environments in which students can be assigned limited numbers of clients and focus intently on the details of assessment, treatment planning, and the "long version" of clinical reporting. ASHA says that a student's initial practicum experiences should be in such a sheltered environment where time can be taken to learn some basics of clinical documentation prior to going to off-campus settings.

Easing the Transition into Clinical Practicum in the University Clinical Setting

As we said in Chapter 1, professionalism is all about communication. It is through communication that you project yourself as a professional whether it is verbally or in writing. It is important that you are proactive in approaching your clinical practicum and do some planning and preparation for the experience. If you are proactive, some of the fear of the unknown will be lessened and you will gain a certain amount of control over events. In some university clinics, you will have just completed undergraduate classes in the normal processes of speech, hearing, and language and some of the disorders courses when you will have the opportunity to engage in clinical practicum. First, you will have the chance to observe assessment and treatment, and then you may be assigned a client or two of your own for which you take primary responsibility. Some of you might be in a training program that reserves all the cases for the graduate students. In that case, you can use our advice when you start clinical practicum on the graduate level. In some cases, however, undergraduate students have an opportunity to take partial responsibility for a case, typically in the areas of language or phonology. The case is usually a child, which limits your practicum experience to a specific group of clients. Assuming that you do engage in clinical practicum as an undergraduate, you will feel a distinct difference as you go from a student who takes classes to one who interacts with clients. You go from reading, listening to lectures, studying, and taking tests to planning, executing, and reporting the expectation that you will act and communicate professionally. It is quite a jump from being a fairly anonymous student in a class of 30 to taking responsibility for a treatment session. So, what advice can we give you to help ease the transition into clinical practicum and make it appear that your professionalism quotient is fairly high? We provide general information below that will prepare you for what you will experience.

The Medical Setting

Figure 2–3 attempts to illustrate the mood of the medical setting. Note that it is considerably different from the university environment. Professionals wear specific clothing, in most cases scrubs, which make everyone from a skilled surgeon to the maintenance personnel look like doctors. Patients, depending on their units, may be wearing hospital gowns or everyday clothes. Some patients are in beds, while others travel using a variety of different devices such as wheelchairs, walkers, and canes. Some patients have equipment such as IV stands or oxygen tanks. There is an obvious emphasis on infection control as evident by a smell of disinfectant and copious boxes of gloves. All of a sudden, you are working with other professionals from physical therapy (PT), occupational therapy (OT), respiratory therapy (RT), and nursing. You get the distinct feeling that you are not in Kansas anymore. In medical settings such as hospitals, rehabilitation centers, and skilled nursing facilities, there is a whole new set of regulatory influences on clinical practice. Whereas ASHA was the "Big Brother" in the university setting, medical environments are under no regulatory constraints from this organization. As indicated in Table 2–1, medical settings are mostly regulated by federal and state hospital guidelines, Medicare, Medicaid, and third-party payers such as insurance companies. These influences will have a direct impact on how long you

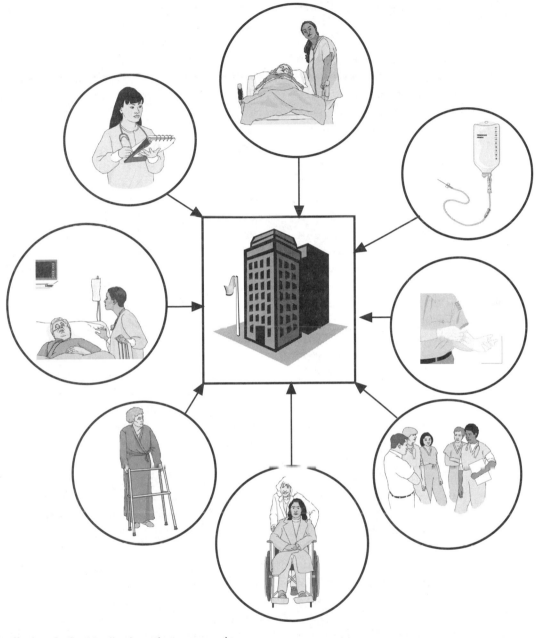

Figure 2–3. Medical settings are unique.

can see your patient, the goals you address, and paperwork associated with medical settings.

With regard to your training, medical settings have the following goals:

■ Expose students to varied caseloads of medically based communication disorders in children and adults.

■ Expose students to the physical facilities common for hospitals, rehabilitation centers, and skilled nursing residences.

■ Expose students to allied professionals (e.g., nurses, certified nursing assistants, nutritionists, physical therapists, occupational therapists, physicians, radiologists) typically encountered in medical settings.

■ Expose students to the unique culture of medical settings with its attendant terminologies, equipment, and paperwork requirements.

When we refer to medical settings in this book, we are including acute care hospitals, inpatient rehabilitation facilities (IRFs), and skilled nursing facilities (SNFs). While these settings have some overlap, they are each unique, and patients' experiences vary according to their diagnoses and payment source. The length of stay (LOS) may average several days in an acute care setting to several weeks in an inpatient rehabilitation facility. Although skilled nursing facilities have some beds designated as "rehab" beds in which patients stay for a period of time before discharging home or elsewhere, patients often remain until the end of their life. Admission criteria to IRFs and SNFs vary, again according to patient status and payment source. Unlike in the university clinic where patients can attend therapy for as long as they wish, therapy is limited to a specific number of sessions or length of time.

When students go to a medical setting for the first time, they are usually in a state of shock. First, the pace is considerably faster in medical settings because there are many more clients who are seen for shorter sessions as compared to the university clinic. In the hospital or rehabilitation environment, everyone is using terminologies that are unique to the medical setting, and students new to this environment are often intimidated by this unique language. Also, you are interacting with other professionals in physical therapy, occupational therapy, respiratory therapy, and nursing, all of whom have their own jargon you have to learn and understand. Patients will be arriving in wheelchairs or using walkers or quad canes. The patients may have just been to physical or occupational therapy and now must battle fatigue to attend and participate in a focused treatment session. Often, the clients the student saw in the university clinic were children with language and phonological disorders, and now the patients are adults who have neurogenically based communication disorders or dysphagia. There will probably be less time spent in supervisory conferences as compared to the university. In some cases, a facility will have a standard protocol for treatment or assessment plans, and very little actual planning will be required of the student beyond how to implement the program. In some settings there may be a standard set of treatment materials in the form of a workbook that the student and client will use.

One of the biggest changes students see in medical settings is the different way of reporting assessment and treatment activity. The most noticeable difference is the brevity of reporting in medical settings. Students will do assessments in 30 minutes, and the "report" may only be a form that includes boxes to check with a few lines available for a narrative sentence or two. Most facilities utilize an electronic medical record. In IRFs, a patient's functional independence measure (FIM) score will mean more to the third-party payers than will your narrative sentences. A patient's length of stay in the facility is dependent upon the numbers the patient is assigned on admission. The patient's chart is a central point of communication in medical settings and the patient's status and progress must be summarized for other professionals to read. This is quite different from the lengthy narrative reports the student has written in university clinics. The chart in the medical setting allows each of the professionals involved in the patient's care to document their interactions with the patient. Charting in these locations can be fairly short and includes pertinent information only. The patient's known case history information, plan of care, physician's orders, nurses' notes, therapist notes, and notes regarding medical exams/procedures are all included in the chart. The chart is kept in a central location, usually the nurses' station, to allow all professionals equal access. While you should omit flowery and verbose descriptions while making chart notes, you should remember the common saying, "If it's not written in the chart, it didn't happen." Therefore, if you do not document that you educated a patient regarding safe swallow strategies and the patient says you did not, you are held accountable for not providing the patient with the information.

Students often complain that one of the most difficult things about professional reporting in the medical setting is learning how to communicate clinical results in a brief and economical format. What took an entire paragraph in a university report might only be communicated in a sentence or phrase in a patient's chart. It is not unusual for students who have completed a rotation in a medical setting to come confidently back into the university clinic in their scrubs and suggest that all of the time and detail spent on clinical reports in the training program were overkill and not reflective of the real world. It is important to remember, however, that before you can scale down information for a medical chart, you have to know what you are talking about. One cannot fully appreciate the elegance of a well-crafted, parsimonious phrase unless exactly how the economical version really does reflect the reality of the patient's progress is understood. We should always remember that checking boxes on an assessment form is often done at the expense of not painting a comprehensive picture of the patient.

Easing the Transition to Medical Practicum Settings

It is important to realize that when you arrive at a new practicum setting, you are not only representing yourself as a burgeoning professional, but you are also acting as a representative of your training program. Thus, it is critical that you think very carefully about the first impression you give to the professionals in your new practicum setting. Remember, the SLPs working in a hospital, rehabilitation center, or nursing facility are true professionals who have their own reputations to consider, as well as the reputation of their unit in the medical setting. Medical settings are divided into a host of different departments such as radiology, psychology, SLP, physical therapy, occupational therapy, and so on. Each unit has its departmental reputation to protect, and each professional working in the department is ultimately responsible for the actions of practicum students they supervise. If you create difficulties or act unprofessionally, it reflects not only on your immediate supervisor, but on that person's department and the university training program as well. So, like it or not, the pressure is on and the ball is in your court. You will remember that we promised to give you some good advice to ease the transition into different practicum settings, so in the next few sections, help is on the way.

We indicated earlier in the chapter that a major purpose of this text is to assist students in developing professional attitudes and behaviors. One way of doing that is to think *proactively* as you move through your clinical practicum. We have tried to illustrate that one stumbling block in your practicum experience might be the differences you will encounter in the various types of work settings to which you are assigned. Knowing that you will have to make some adjustments in how you act and perform various tasks should be a first step to regaining control. It is important that you do some thinking and planning before you arrive at a strange practicum site. Be prepared to present yourself as a professional in training who has certain competencies but has come to the medical setting to learn more. Obviously, you are not coming to the hospital setting because you are a seasoned veteran who knows what to do. You have some knowledge from classes, and you might have even worked with some clients in the university clinic who have medically related communication disorders. But, this may be your first experience with medical SLP. Whatever your situation, you can still make a good first impression on your new practicum supervisor(s). It is critical, however, that you not merely waltz into the hospital and say, "I'm here!" Adequate preparation on your part will make all the difference when meeting your supervisors for the first time. Following are some areas you might consider in planning your first visit to a new practicum site:

1. **Prepracticum visit:** When possible, we recommend that instead of just showing up on your first day of scheduled practicum, you meet with your supervisor ahead of time. We understand that this may not always be feasible; however, it shows that you are interested, serious minded, and professional. At times, the medical facility may request this meeting before you do to discuss their policies, but regardless of who makes the appointment, it is a good tactic to make a prepracticum visit. Typically, you will be assigned to one supervisor but you would be prudent to ask at your meeting if you will be rotating among several supervisors or shadowing the same one throughout your practicum.

2. **Orientation:** During your prepracticum visit you should ask about any orientation that will be provided by the facility for new practicum students. Again, your new supervisor may be planning to introduce this topic, but if she does not, you should ask. If the supervisor begins by telling you about a mandatory orientation meeting, you can say, "Good. That was one of the things I was going to ask about, and I'm so glad that an orientation is available." Orientations are frequently required before your internship for the purpose of educating you about privacy laws and policies, infection control, and specific facility protocols.

3. **Being honest about your training:** Although practicum supervisors may see many students from university training programs, the students may have different levels of experience in medical SLP. It is important that you are honest about knowledge and experience, it is fine to tell your new supervisor what you feel comfortable with and in which areas you still have a lot to learn. It is especially important to communicate your interest in learning new things and that you appreciate the opportunity to learn as much as possible during your practicum experience. Supervisors do not expect you to "know it all," just be willing to try and be receptive to instruction and suggestions.

4. **Learn names and the organizational structure:** Obviously, it is important for you to write down the names of any people you will be interacting with on a daily basis in the practicum placement. Do not be afraid to jot down those names because it is not unusual for you to meet many people during a visit including the SLP staff, people from other disciplines (physical therapy, occupational therapy, physicians, nurses), patients, hospital administrators, secretarial staff, and other practicum students. It makes a good impression when you return if you can remember the names of people you met during your visit. Perhaps even more important than remembering names is figuring out the organizational structure of the facility in which you will be working. Like any organization, medical facilities have a power structure that is important to learn if you are going to be working there. For example, the SLP unit may be composed of three SLPs, one of whom has administrative responsibility over the department. The speech-pathology unit may be part of a larger department that includes physical therapy, occupational therapy, respiratory therapy, and some other types of allied health professions. There is an administrator who oversees all of these different types of therapy and the SLP coordinator has to answer to this person. Our point here is that it is important for you to see where you are in the organizational arrangement of your medical facility and who is in charge at various levels. You never know when you will need to work with other departments and general offices such as risk management, security, or administrative offices. Your supervisor will be the person to inform you regarding these matters.

5. **Handouts:** It is appropriate for you to ask about the availability of any orientation handouts or brochures that cover policies and procedures of the facility in general and the SLP section in particular. Many practicum sites have informative manuals they have constructed just for practicum students to orient them to the setting. It is almost impossible for you to write down everything you are told in a prepracticum visit, so asking for a handout shows that you are interested in and serious about adhering to the rules and guidelines of the facility.

6. **Your schedule:** It is important to ask specific questions about your schedule such as when to arrive each day, where to report when you arrive, where to park, and when to leave. You cannot be punctual if you do not know your schedule. This would be a good time to have your supervisor describe a typical day you might experience, from start to finish. You should also ask about special events that will concern you (e.g., accreditation visits, hospital or department meetings). Please remember that flexibility is key, especially in medical settings where you are treating sick people. It is likely that some days you may have to stay longer than your scheduled time to finish your work for the day. In most cases, your schedule will mirror that of your assigned supervisor, so if he or she is staying late, you will be expected to as well.

7. **Responsibilities:** This is also a good time to ask about your responsibilities as a practicum student and how they might change as you gain more experience. You should ask about supervision in terms of how frequently it is provided and the opportunities for supervisory conferences regarding your

caseload. Asking about the evaluation process that will be used to grade your clinical work would also be appropriate at this time. It is possible that in some settings you will not see patients without supervision in the beginning. You may be observing or working with your supervising SLP at first. The supervisor can tell you how they work with practicum students, and you should be interested in this. It would be good to know that during a practicum experience, greater responsibility will gradually be shifted to you as you progress in the training.

8. **The facilities:** Ask for a tour of the facilities and where you will be seeing patients for assessment and treatment. Will you go to a dedicated room? Will you see some patients in their hospital room? Will you be working with groups? Where will group therapy be held? Will you be co-treating with professionals from other disciplines?

9. **Transport:** Medical facilities have various regulations about transporting patients. Some patients in wheelchairs are often transported from one therapy to another by aides and sometimes by the person who just finished treating them (such as physical therapist). The point here is that you should be aware of what the conventions are in the facility and how patients get from one place to another. Also, be aware that, while it may not be your job to transport a patient to therapy, you may be required to do this in the event that other personnel are busy. A major issue involves transferring patients from beds to wheelchairs, or vice versa. You should not do this without specific training because of possible injury to the patient or yourself. Find out the procedures

that are used in your facility before you start working with patients, or else you could make a big mistake.

10. **Paperwork:** Because you will be required to produce many reports, notes, and other forms of paperwork, it is only logical that you should have the opportunity to look at examples of such output. In some cases, your supervisor will give you examples with identifying information deleted to protect confidentiality. In other cases, you may be given an opportunity to study patient charts in the office. Whatever the case, it is good to familiarize yourself with the types of paperwork you will be asked to generate so that you can come closer to hitting the mark the first try.

11. **Confidentiality:** Ask about how patient confidentiality is handled at the facility. How is paperwork stored and secured? Are there secure computers available on which to do your reports? Is there a specific way in which you are required to communicate confidential information to others? What disposal methods (shredding, erasing) are available for reports (electronic or paper)?

The School Setting

In Figure 2–4 we try to capture some of the environment of the school setting. The professionals you interact with are regular education teachers, learning disabilities (LD) teachers, special educators, psychologists, special education coordinators, school administrators, and various support personnel. Children attend classes that focus on literacy, content areas of math, science, history, and social studies, and physical education. The classroom is an important milieu, and you hear bells signaling the transition

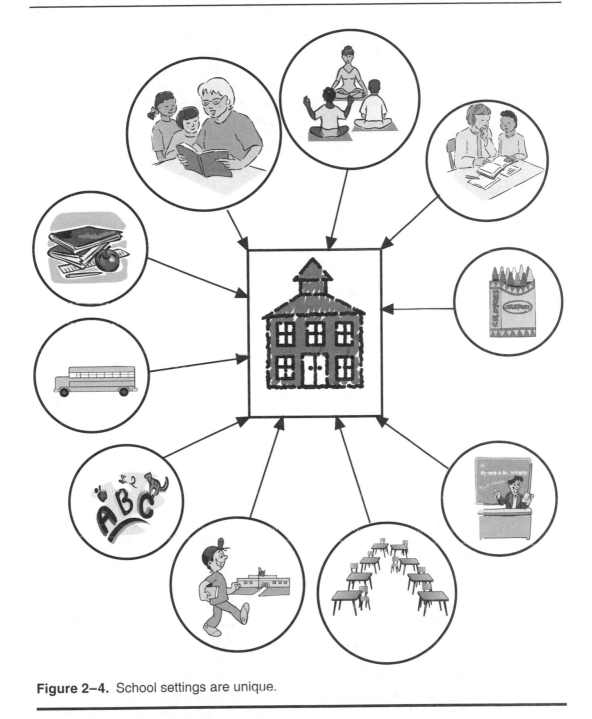

Figure 2–4. School settings are unique.

of one class to another or recess or lunch-time. Placement in a school setting also has unique goals in your clinical training. Just as the university clinic and medical setting offer a special dimension to your education, school systems provide yet another facet to your developing skills. Some of the following are goals of the school setting related to your training:

- Expose students to the varied caseload of the public schools ranging from preschool to adolescence. These caseloads can range from relatively simple disorders of articulation and language to very complex problems involving dysphagia, augmentative communication, head injury, voice disorders, and stuttering.
- Expose students to the physical facilities typically seen in school settings from preschool programs to secondary schools.
- Expose students to allied professionals (e.g., teachers, special educators, psychologists, aides, administrators) typically encountered in the school setting.
- Expose students to the culture of the educational setting with its attendant terminology, equipment, and paperwork requirements.

One thing that is immediately noticeable is that children are being seen for treatment in small groups, as well as individually. The school SLP may also do therapy within the classroom context and incorporate curriculum materials into treatment activities. As indicated in Table 2–1, schools are primarily regulated by federal and state departments of education. There are a series of laws that dictate how business is conducted in school systems ranging from the Individuals with Disabilities Education Act (IDEA) to Section 504 of the Rehabilitation Act and the Americans with Disabilities Act (ADA). These guidelines will be discussed in later chapters; however, they are mentioned here to illustrate that schools are controlled by a myriad of legal guidelines coming from the state and federal governments. Caseloads in the schools are typically high, which makes group therapy a more efficient way of providing services. School systems have very systematic procedures, just as medical facilities do for identifying clients and providing treatment. Specific forms, such as the *Individualized Education Program* (IEP), are standard fare in school systems, and we will talk more about these in a later chapter. Services are provided free of charge, which is a major difference from most other settings. Unfortunately, although the law says that every student should be provided adequate treatment, some school systems may be underfunded and not have enough personnel or facilities to service every child ideally. Other systems have state-of-the-art facilities, a full complement of highly qualified faculty, and small caseloads. Just as hospital settings vary in size, quality, and in terms of personnel, school systems do as well. Remember that school systems must service children from ages 3 to 21, and many districts are providing assessment and treatment from birth onward. School systems use a variety of models to provide services including direct therapy, group therapy, consultative, center-based, and home-based programs. Thus, your practicum experience in the school environment can be quite varied. In the past, the stereotype of a school system was that the caseload was largely made up of language and articulation cases. Today, schools represent one of the most diverse caseload environments available in clinical practice. It is not unusual to see children with head injury, unique syndromes, stuttering, voice disorders, cerebral palsy, autism, swallowing problems, cochlear implants, and hearing impairments. There may be children in the regular classroom who are nonverbal and use an augmentative communication device. Many of the children have been diagnosed with learning disabilities, attention deficit disorder, psychological difficulties, and behavior problems. Thus, the school environment is different from medical or university settings, and this uniqueness is seen in assessment, treatment, reporting, and every other aspect of clinical work.

Easing the Transition to School Practicum Settings

Just as we urged you to be proactive in transitioning into your first practicum case in the university clinic and your introduction to a medical setting, we again suggest planning for your first visit to a school placement. Many of the principles we suggested for the other two settings also apply to practicum in the schools, and we do not provide as much detail here:

1. **Prepracticum visit:** As in the medical setting, we recommend that you visit the school setting prior to your first day of practicum so that you can ask questions and receive instructions from your supervisor.
2. **Orientation:** In some school systems there will be an orientation provided for new practicum students. Be sure to ask about this and attend if it is offered.
3. **Be honest about your training:** In the school system you have a higher likelihood of working with children who have language and phonological disorders. This, in some ways, might be similar to your experience at the university clinic. You will have a larger comfort zone with these clients than you will have with medically oriented disorders in a hospital setting. Thus,

you should feel a bit more comfortable in the school setting. Share with your practicum supervisor the types of experiences you have had in the university clinic and those cases in which you are particularly interested.

4. **Learn names and the organizational structure:** As in the medical setting, there will be many names for you to learn in the school placement: the SLP(s), school nurse, school psychologist, many regular classroom teachers, special education teachers, learning disabilities specialists, reading teachers, school administrators such as principals and assistant principals, a special education coordinator, and the secretarial staff. To compound this, you will often be assigned to multiple school buildings and so the names increase exponentially. The school organizational structure is both similar to and different from the medical setting. Schools tend to have a superintendent who oversees the entire school system. Each school is run administratively by a principal and assistant principal who control what happens in their building. An SLP is typically under a special education coordinator who might oversee psychology, SLP, learning disabilities, special education, and reading disabilities. Thus, although you might be supervised by an SLP, you both may be ultimately responsible to the special education coordinator. Depending on the size of the school system, there might actually be an SLP department composed of many SLPs, and one is designated as the head of the department. No matter where you are assigned, it is important to note where you fit into the organizational structure and to whom you are responsible.

5. **Handouts:** If the school system has any handouts on its policies, it is a good idea to obtain these and become familiar with them prior to your practicum. There may also be handouts generated by the SLP department that are designed for practicum students.

6. **Your schedule:** Like any work setting, there will be expectations regarding when you will arrive for work, when you can leave, and where you will go during the work day. School systems often have employees sign in and out of school buildings. You should ask specifically about your typical daily schedule and any special events (e.g., assemblies, staffings, IEP meetings) that you will be expected to attend.

7. **Responsibilities:** As in the medical setting, your supervisor might start you off with limited responsibilities and increase them as you gain more experience. You should ask about your initial responsibilities and how they are likely to change over time. This would be a good time to ask about the caseload you will be working with in terms of types of disorders, severity, and frequency of therapy. You should also ask if you are seeing the children individually, in groups, or in the classroom setting. This allows you to anticipate the types of activities you will need to prepare for treatment.

8. **Facilities:** You will want to know where you will be working with children in the school. Is there a dedicated speech pathology room complete with materials? Is most of the treatment done in the classroom setting? Are you sharing a room with other professionals?

9. **Transport:** It is important to determine how the children will get to your treatment sessions. Will you go to the class-room and escort them to therapy? Will the children of a certain age be trusted to come to therapy by themselves? Will the teacher remind them?

10. **Paperwork:** The school system has unique paperwork compared to other settings. You will need to become familiar with IEPs and individual family service plans (IFSPs) and many other forms generated by the school system. It would be helpful if you could obtain example copies of such forms with identifying information removed so that you can approximate these models in your initial attempts at generating paperwork. Even though you will not be totally responsible for writing them, you will want to become familiar with forms used in the school setting. We discuss these in later chapters and reference online examples.

11. **Confidentiality:** In all settings you will be required to maintain confidentiality about your clients. You should ask about this issue in the school setting and determine how information is safeguarded and disposed of when no longer needed.

This chapter aimed to introduce you to aspects of your upcoming clinical practicum that students rarely contemplate. Most students think of their practicum experience as a unified, seamless progression that is part of their clinical training. They rarely realize that there are unavoidable adjustments and bumps in the road that will make them question their abilities and the wisdom of those who designed their training program. Hopefully, this chapter has demonstrated to you that moving from one practicum site to another invariably means adjusting what you know and learning new approaches to old problems. The inevitability of having to make adjustments to different practicum settings allows you to anticipate these bumps in the road and take proactive steps to make the transition a bit more comfortable. The following chapters are designed to help you plan for different practicum placements and their attendant diverse environments, approaches to clinical work, and demands for professional communication.

3

Ethics, Confidentiality, and Safeguarding Clinical Communications

The field of speech-language pathology (SLP) is as diverse as it is dynamic and serves a large population of clients. This, in turn, makes speech pathology a public service. Those in the field recognize that the well-being of the people we serve comes first. To that end, confidentiality and safeguarding all information regarding our clients and patients are paramount.

Due to modern technology, public as well as private information is more accessible than ever before. As a result, identity theft and fraudulent use of confidential information have become commonplace. The need for guidelines to ensure the confidentiality of patients under any doctor or specialist's care was recognized not only by the health care providers themselves but also by the federal government.

In 1996, President Bill Clinton signed the Health Information Portability and Accountability Act, or HIPAA, also known as Public Law 104-191. One of the provisions of HIPAA was to establish measures that ensure the security and privacy of health care information maintained by health care providers, both public and private.

How this relates to speech pathology encompasses many things. Private practices, hospitals, rehabilitation facilities, and long-term care facilities have many forms of communication that contain patient information. Most of this information is viewed by a diverse group of people involved in the patient's care. As a result, the speech-language pathologist may discuss patient and client issues with other relevant professionals on a daily basis. Referrals to other agencies may be made, resulting in information being passed via mail or electronically. It is imperative that the patient's information is protected so that abuse of any kind does not occur.

In addition, clients and caregivers have a legal right to read any report containing information about themselves or their family members (Family Educational Rights & Privacy Act of 1974, Public Law 93-380 [FERPA]). To this end, providers of SLP services must be accountable, not only in keeping accurate data regarding progress made in therapy, but in protecting the privacy of the clients they serve. Another fun fact about FERPA is how it impacts students. You would be surprised at how many calls your professors receive from concerned parents who want to know how you are doing in classes. According to the law, we cannot discuss student performance without your expressed permission. So, even though you might not have known about it, your privacy is being protected by the law. We hope, of course, that you are proud of your performance and share it with your parents, but it is your right to keep them in the dark, if you so desire.

ASHA Code of Ethics

As professionals who are governed by a licensing board, we also have an ethical responsibility to our clients and patients. The American Speech-Language-Hearing Association (ASHA) has a code of ethics (ASHA, 2010) just as other professional organizations such as psychology, medicine, nursing, occupational therapy, education, and physical therapy prescribe ethical responsibilities of practitioners. We do not want to turn this chapter into a review of the entire Code of Ethics, but would like to mention certain ethical issues that address professional communication.

Several portions of the ASHA Code of Ethics relate to the notions of professionalism and communication. We quote these directly from the 2010 version of the Code of Ethics, and you should be able to see how they relate to *professionalism* and *communication* (ASHA, 2010):

- "Individuals shall not reveal, without authorization, any professional or personal information about identified persons served professionally or identified participants involved in research and

scholarly activities unless doing so is necessary to protect the welfare of the person or of the community, or is otherwise required by law" (Principle of Ethics I, Rule N).

- "Individuals shall fully inform the persons they serve of the nature and possible effects of services rendered and products dispensed, and they shall inform participants in research about the possible effects of their participation in research conducted" (Principle of Ethics I, Rule H).

- "Individuals shall not guarantee the results of any treatment or procedure, directly or by implication; however, they may make a reasonable statement of prognosis" (Principle of Ethics I, Rule J).

- "Individuals shall not misrepresent their credentials, competence, education, training, experience, or scholarly or research contributions" (Principle of Ethics III, Rule A).

- "Individuals shall not misrepresent research, diagnostic information, services rendered, results of services rendered, products dispensed or the effects of products dispensed" (Principle of Ethics III, Rule D).

- "Individuals' statements to the public shall provide accurate information about the nature and management of communication disorders, about the professions, about professional services, about products for sale, and about research and scholarly activities" (Principle of Ethics III, Rule F).

- "Individuals' statements to the public when advertising, announcing, and marketing their professional services; reporting research results; and promoting products shall adhere to professional standards and shall not contain misrepresentations" (Principle of Ethics III, Rule G).

- ▪ "Individuals shall not engage in dishonesty, fraud, deceit, or misrepresentation" (Principle of Ethics IV, Rule C).
- ▪ "Individuals' statements to colleagues about professional services, research results, and products shall adhere to prevailing professional standards and shall contain no misrepresentations" (Principle of Ethics IV, Rule I).

The word *professional* appears in almost all of these ethical guidelines. Note that almost all of them include the notion of "communication" either explicitly or implicitly. Many of the statements have a great deal to do with the idea that an SLP is expected to communicate with colleagues and patients accurately, in a professional manner, without misrepresenting his or her clinical practice. Even in our advertising we must meet "professional standards" and not place an advertisement as if we were selling used automobiles. It is no coincidence that announcements and advertising from many different professions (e.g., physicians, dentists, psychologists) all look similar. Thus, we hope you can see that our Code of Ethics places a great deal of emphasis on professional communication. In the next few sections we will zero in on the notion of confidentiality in both written and verbal professional communication across work settings.

The University Speech and Hearing Clinic

The university speech and hearing clinic will be your first foray into dealing with confidential clinical information and acting

with a degree of professionalism. If you are not already aware of it, all of our clients deserve the right to privacy in seeking clinical services. Most, if not all, SLP graduate programs now require HIPAA training for incoming graduate students, as well as faculty and staff who provide clinical services. We have worked with adult clients who have specifically requested that they not be observed by students in our training program. Although we would like to give students the opportunity to view all treatment sessions, we have to respect the rights of our clients to their privacy. Some clients request privacy only in the beginning of treatment, and then as they gain expertise in communication they are proud of their accomplishments and welcome observers.

George Adams was a retired history professor whose progressive Parkinson's disease essentially put a stop to his teaching career. He had an extremely tremulous voice and made uncontrolled upper body movements even sitting in a chair. Because Dr. Adams had taught at the university for 40 years, he came to the speech and hearing clinic for services. He had only retired a year ago, so he was concerned that some of his former students would still be around to see the ravages of Parkinson's disease on his appearance and communication. He specifically requested that no students be allowed to observe his treatment sessions.

Michael (Michelle) Jenrette had made a most drastic decision. He had decided to begin the process of sexual reassignment and become a woman. This very personal decision was not made lightly and Mr. Jenrette had undergone extensive counseling from physicians and psychologists. As part of his transition from male to female he had to learn new vocal production patterns, nonverbal communication, and language structures common to women.

> Mr. Jenrette was a faculty member at the university, and he had not yet shared his decision with coworkers or even some of his family members. Thus, it was important for the speech and hearing clinic staff to maintain confidentiality and not talk openly about this case. Mr. Jenrette also requested that no one observe his treatment sessions.

There are multiple opportunities for breaches in confidentiality to arise in the university training program. First, we generate reams of paperwork related to assessment, treatment, and student training. Second, much of this paperwork is handled on a daily basis by students who have never been responsible for protecting the personal privacy of clients. In the university speech clinic, sources of personal information include, but are not limited to

- Daily notes and treatment plans
- Formal treatment reports
- Formal diagnostic reports
- Information on flash drives
- Electronic transmissions (faxes, e-mails, billing)
- Authorization forms signed by clients
- Therapy schedules
- Verbal discussions
- Video/audio recordings

Each of these is discussed in more detail below.

Treatment Plans and Progress Notes

The treatment plan and progress note are vital to the SLP's daily routine in a university clinic. The treatment plan details the clinician's specific plan for the session, which may include the goals to be targeted and the procedures, cues, and reinforcement that will be implemented. In the university clinic, the student writes a treatment plan prior to the session and a progress note after the session. The progress note provides accountability for what takes places in the clinical session through the documentation of data collection, assessment of a client's performance, and plans for future sessions. Both notes may be kept in a client file separate from the permanent record, or if the clinic uses a computer system to manage client information, the treatment plan and progress note will be stored electronically. These files should only be accessible to clinicians and supervisors as part of the safeguarding procedure. The progress note and treatment plan may contain less personal information about the client, as the student may use a client's file number, date of birth, or initials as identifying information; however, if any form is no longer needed, it should be shredded rather than thrown anyway. No client information should leave the clinic at any point.

Formal Treatment Reports

The formal treatment report includes identifying information, data, and a summary of client performance that usually covers one semester. These reports include a great deal of personal information about a client such as name, date of birth, address, telephone number, referring physician, diagnosis, and so forth. It is important that this information is not handled casually and that the student or students who are working with this client do not leave these reports in public areas or open on a computer screen where anyone can read this confidential information. In our university's clinic, computers that students use are password protected and in a locked area that is not accessible to the public.

Copy Confusion

Carmen Jones was in a hurry. Her treatment reports on five clients were due to be turned in to her supervisor in less than an hour. She needed to make three copies of each report for distribution to the client folder, parents, and the school system. Carmen found an open Xerox machine at the local copying store and placed each of her five reports in the feeder tray, pressing the appropriate buttons for three copies each. As the copies came out, Carmen paper-clipped them together in a pile and removed the original from the machine. When the last copy was done, she looked at her watch and realized that she had only 10 minutes to get to the clinic. As Carmen grabbed all her copies and rushed out the door, she was oblivious to the fact that the original from the last report she had copied remained in the document feeder. The next person to use that machine would have a golden opportunity to learn about Tyrone Walker, an elementary school student with autism whose mother places a high value on privacy.

Formal Diagnostic Reports

Just as with the formal treatment report, the diagnostic report also contains a great deal of personal information about a client. In fact, the diagnostic report is likely to contain the *most* personal information of any of our professional communications. By their very nature, diagnostic reports contain a plethora of historical information, not only about the client, but the family as well. So, if a child exhibits behavior problems, such as bed-wetting or thumb-sucking, it is all laid out in the case history. If a child has developed disfluencies since his parents' divorce, it is noted in the historical section of the report. Also included in the case history might be test scores from other professionals who have evaluated the client previously. Some of these, such as IQ scores, are noted in the case history and constitute very sensitive information. If a client is being seen by another professional (e.g., psychologist, physician), this is outlined in the case history. The diagnostic report also includes all of the test results of the SLP evaluation including standard scores and percentile ranks of performance on various assessment instruments. Finally, the report will include the evaluator's interpretation of the test results and the formal diagnosis of a disorder. This report may also include recommendations for referrals to other professionals in addition to a diagnosis and prognosis. It is easy to see that no one would want such personal information to be compromised. Our clients assume that any information they divulge will be treated with confidentiality, and a professional should treat this obligation very seriously.

Rainy Day Reporting

Susan Pierce arrived at the university speech and hearing clinic parking lot just in time to grab the last parking space available. It was a rainy Monday morning and she was not looking forward to her back-to-back schedule of supervisory conferences with speech pathology practicum students. Susan had been a clinical supervisor for 5 years and thought she had "seen it all" with regard to student problems. Struggling to open her umbrella and exit her car at the same time, she immediately stepped into a large puddle adjacent to the driver's side door. It was then that she noticed the paper that was pinned squarely in the water beneath her fashionable black high-heeled pump. Through the water she read the smudged yet legible clinic letterhead; and under that was the section called "Identifying Information," which contained the client's name, address, telephone, and other personal information. Further down was a section devoted to case history, which described the devastation in the wake of a major stroke and the effects on the client's job and family. Although the type was a bit smeared, it was easy to read all the sensitive personal information that had been given in confidence to a caring clinician. Literally hundreds of people pass through this parking lot in a day, and Susan could only speculate how many of them might have paused to read this lost report. As you might anticipate, every report is signed by the student clinician and supervisor, and Susan's heart sank as she observed her own name at the bottom of the second page. This grim scenario probably began as an innocent lapse in safeguarding confidential information with a partially zipped backpack, unsnapped notebook, or papers being blown unobserved from the front seat of a vehicle. But innocent or not, such lapses in safeguarding information have repercussions and consequences. The chain of events can affect the client, the supervisor, the reputation of the clinic, and the perception of the student. Susan strode into the building, her lips drawn back into a thin red line, hoping she would see the student clinician responsible for this unforgivable breakdown in protecting client confidentiality.

Information on Flash Drives Used by Students

Many students maintain information about their client(s) on flash drives in order to keep track of the information more efficiently. Students should be very cautious about using flash drives in computers outside of the university clinic or their own personal computers. It is not uncommon for a student to have his or her "whole life" on that one flash drive, such as personal correspondence, classroom work, term papers,

and drafts of clinical reports as well. The reason manufacturers put lanyards on those flash drives is that they are likely to be lost or misplaced because of their compact size. If you lose your flash drive you are not only losing your whole life but the lives of any clients who are mentioned in those files. In order to ensure that your client's privacy is protected while you have his or her reports on a flash drive, you should not use any identifying information. This may include representing the client's name with initials or a file number or otherwise deleting any confidential personal information. If you keep any electronic copies of your reports, make sure they are in a safe place; even better, delete those files after the information is no longer of use.

The Hard Lesson of the Hard Drive

Candace Newman was a master of using time between classes to do her homework. If she had a free hour, she would go to one of the 10 student computer labs located across the large university campus. It was a great opportunity to work on term papers for core classes in English, history, sociology, and science. It was also a chance to work on clinical reports for several clients she was seeing in practicum at the university speech and hearing clinic. Candace had diagnostic reports and midterm treatment reports that were due to be turned in to her supervisor within a week. With only 5 minutes remaining before her next class, Candace hurriedly saved her document. She had done so much work on the report that she decided to check her personal computer disk to see if the document had actually been saved. When she looked at the directory for her disk, the report was not there. So she saved the report again and confirmed that it was, in fact, on her disk. Unknown to Candace, however, her first attempt at saving the report ended up on the public computer's hard drive. Now the report, which detailed the history and personal information of Joey Dean, a child with fragile X syndrome, was available in a public computer lab for anyone to access. Maybe no one would pull the document up at all and the information would be lost in the maw of files on the hard drive. On the other hand, maybe someone would be curious about the file and access it to see what it was. Either way, Candace has planted a confidentiality time bomb that might come back to haunt her, the university clinic, her supervisor, and worst of all, Joey's family. Only time will tell.

Electronic Transmissions

Much of the communication between the university clinic and outside referral sources, allied health professionals, students and instructors, and even clients may be communicated via electronic mail (e-mail). Clinic personnel, as well as student clinicians, should be aware that this information may be read by someone other than the person or persons for whom it was intended. To this end, any and all attempts to protect our clients' privacy should be made. Identifying information such as file numbers or initials may be used instead of a client's name. More commonly now, your university may have a program in place that allows supervisors and students to transfer confidential information by encrypting the files.

Authorization Forms

Most university clinics require clients to sign an authorization form, or "release" in order to evaluate and/or provide speech therapy services. This form is usually kept in the client's confidential file, and therefore is not subject to viewing by anyone other than clinic staff. At some university clinics that have a sliding fee schedule, prospective clients are required to report information on family size and personal income to qualify for reduced fees. Such financial information is obviously very sensitive and must be safeguarded.

Therapy Schedules

At our clinic, a comprehensive schedule of all client appointments is located on a computer in the student clinicians' room. This room requires swipe access by students and faculty, and the computer program is password protected; therefore, confidential client information is not accessible to individuals who are not associated with the clinic. The students are alerted to their client's arrival or cancellation via the computer.

Verbal Discussions

In a university setting it is not uncommon for students to communicate with one another in classes, before classes, while waiting for a client to arrive, or just walking down a corridor in the speech and hearing clinic. One of the things our students have in common is their experiences in classes and in clinical practicum. Thus, it may seem natural to discuss a client you are working with, especially if you are having a great deal of success, are frustrated due to lack of progress, or just experienced something funny during your session. While you are having these conversations you never know who will be in a position to overhear what you say. Treatment rooms are typically close to clinician areas, resulting in limited privacy and requiring you to take great care to use a volume that is appropriate and be aware of your surroundings when you are discussing clients. Although you should maintain client confidentiality by not revealing identifying information, it is okay to ask about certain procedures or goals during your academic classes. This gives you an opportunity to share with your classmates and to ensure that you understand why you are doing what you are doing.

Foot in Mouth Disease

Toni and Trisha were standing by the restroom in the clinic hallway talking about one of their clients who had not had a very productive session.

"He can be a real brat!" Trisha complained.

"Yeah, he was terrible today. I'm sure glad I don't have to take him home," Toni replied.

Trisha laughed as she sipped her Diet Coke. "And can you believe his mother thinks he doesn't have a behavior problem? What's up with that?"

About that time, the mother walks out of the restroom and into the hall where the students are standing. Trisha almost chokes on her Diet Coke, as Toni, red faced, picks up her cell phone and begins a text message to her boyfriend. Mom turns and walks down the hall, obviously hurt by their rude remarks. The students look at each other in disbelief. "Wow, we really messed up that time," Toni mumbles.

The next week, the mother calls the clinic and cancels her son's therapy appointment. Then, she cancels the next one, and the next one, until it's almost mid-semester. Finally, when the clinical supervisor calls to ask her if there's a problem, she says, "Yes, there certainly is, your students were saying terrible things about me and my son and I don't appreciate it one bit. I'll never come back to that clinic!"

Students should also be aware that the danger of being overheard lurks outside the clinic environment as well. When you are at the mall, at a restaurant, in a nightclub, or at church you might be tempted to discuss your clinical work with a friend. If you use identifying information in these conversations there is always a chance that your client's friend, neighbor, coworker, teacher, or relative might just be at the adjacent table or strolling behind you in the mall. This is especially dangerous in small communities where people tend to know everything that is going on. *Thus, a good rule of thumb is if you have any doubt about whether to discuss information about a client, then don't.*

Audio/Video Recordings

Recording sessions are useful for accurate data collection, analysis with your supervisor, self-evaluation, or client feedback. Students may be expected to provide their own device to record; however, most clinics offer additional resources. Small digital recorders are relatively inexpensive and easy to place close to your client. Although the sound quality is typically not as good, video recording may be beneficial to glean additional detail from your sessions, especially with certain disorders. Each observation room in our clinic has a DVD player with the capability to record to the hard drive or to a CD for later review. Whether you are using a video recorder, audio recorder, or technology such as an iPad, you will need to take steps to protect your client's privacy. When listening to the recording for the purpose of data collection or analysis with your supervisor, you should choose a private environment that allows for limited access of persons not involved with your case. It is vital that after you have used the sample to gather data or use for client feedback that you delete the recording from the respective device.

In this part of the chapter, we have been discussing confidentiality as it applies to the university clinic. The next sections discuss the issue of confidentiality as it relates to medical and school settings.

The Medical Setting

There are a number of medical settings in which speech/language evaluation and treatment take place: hospitals, long-term care facilities, skilled nursing facilities, and rehabilitation hospitals, to name a few. In our field, the term *medical setting* is generally used to refer to institutions that treat patients who have been diagnosed with any type of illness, injury, disease, or other condition that affects their speech, language, or swallowing function. These facilities are normally staffed by medical personnel such as doctors, nurses, therapists, and various other specialists. In general, a university clinic, public school, or private practice is not considered a medical setting due to the absence of any medically trained personnel.

However, there are exceptions, in that some university clinics are associated with teaching hospitals and therefore may consult with physicians or other medical professionals.

Most of the paperwork that contains client information in a medical setting is similar to paperwork seen in the university clinic (i.e., evaluation reports, therapy plans, progress notes, SOAP notes). In the university setting or private practice, each patient has a file or chart that is typically kept in the clinic office or stored electronically, and the only professional who contributes to the chart is the SLP or audiologist. In medical facilities, the patient's chart is kept in a controlled central location so that the many different professionals involved in the patient's care can have access to it. It is paramount that this information is kept confidential. It is also not a good idea to discuss a patient with anyone other than those involved in the patient's care. Often, a patient in a medical setting is noncommunicative and is therefore at the mercy of a caregiver or facility staff to protect his or her privacy. In this case, the student clinician should be aware of the responsibility to protect the rights of the patient. Any violation of these rights is a direct violation of HIPAA and may result in fines, imprisonment, or both. Being regulated by HIPAA means that you must always be conscious of the *who*, *what*, *where*, and *when*: know *who* you can talk to, *what* you can talk about, *where* you can talk about it, and *when* it is appropriate to talk about it.

John Jacobs was a distinguished attorney who had a stroke in the middle of a trial while defending his client for a murder he did not commit. Right in the middle of his introductory remarks he slumped over the table and the bailiff called 911. As a result of his stroke, Mr. Jacobs could not talk at all but could think as clearly as ever. He was incontinent and forced to wear a hospital gown that was open in the back. People he did not know wandered in and out of his room with various missions involving respiration, speech, meals, and changing IVs. He was poked and prodded by everyone from social workers to student nurses. He had a roommate who continually turned the shared television up so loud that there was no time for personal reflection. So, here was John Jacobs, attorney-at-law, who had lost every last vestige of his personal privacy. But there was one more indignity to suffer. He began to cry as he listened to a conversation between two nursing students there to change his catheter. They talked about his personal history, his son who never visited, and even the client accused of murder who was ultimately convicted.

The School Setting

The paperwork in the public schools differs significantly from the medical setting, university clinic, or private practice. This is due, in part, to the nature of the delivery of services, as well as to the federal laws that govern public schools and how they serve students with disabilities.

The Education of all Handicapped Children Act (EHA), also known as Public Law or PL 94-142, passed in 1975, mandated that all handicapped children between the ages of 3 and 21 receive a free, public education appropriate to their need, and in the least restrictive environment. In 1990, as part of its reauthorization by Congress, this law was renamed the Individuals with Disabilities Education Act or IDEA (PL 101-476). To that end, any child with a diagnosed communication disorder is covered under IDEA and entitled to free and appropriate individualized services (Haynes, Moran, & Pindzola, 2006).

Before a child can receive any special education services, including speech-language therapy, an extensive evaluation procedure is required. Once this evaluation process is complete, and it is determined that the child is eligible for special education services, an *Individualized Education Program* (IEP) must be written to meet the needs of the child. Any child with a communication disorder, who is receiving speech therapy services, will have an IEP. The IEP is unique to the school setting and is the cornerstone of a quality education for each child with a disability (U.S. Department of Education, 2005).

In most school settings, the original copy of the IEP is kept in the student's confidential file in an administrative office. Copies of the IEP are usually kept by each teacher or professional who serves the student in the special education capacity, to ensure that all of the student's goals are being addressed.

Parents may, at any time, request a copy of the IEP, at which time the school must provide such. The parent may also request that the school release a copy of the IEP to other professionals who are working with the child, such as a university speech clinic. This is the case with many of our clients, as they are receiving services from their schools as well as at our clinic. As a speech pathology practicum student in the public schools, you will be expected to implement the goals outlined for each student with whom you are assigned to work. The school SLP will usually provide a copy of the student's IEP for you to follow. For more information, go to the Department of Education website (http://idea.ed.gov/explore/view/p/,root,dynamic,TopicalBrief,10,) for a detailed description of the law.

What is important to know regarding ethics and confidentiality is that any failure to implement the goals outlined in the student's IEP is a violation of federal law; therefore, each person who works with a student who has an IEP is accountable for the goals outlined therein, and this information is kept in a confidential space within the school building. Copies of a student's IEP should not be found floating around the school, or even worse, leaving the building.

Public school SLPs also keep many records in addition to the IEP. Each child will have a folder that includes various test results, treatment progress reports, weekly notes, and other forms of confidential information such as audio/video recordings. This information must be safeguarded as in any other setting until it is disposed of using appropriate methods.

We have tried to illustrate in the present chapter that there is an intimate relationship between professional ethics, protecting confidentiality, and professional communication. These relationships cross work settings and are *always* an important factor in the daily conduct of clinical work. Thus, as a student moving from one setting to another you will always carry with you a concern about patient privacy and confidentiality. It is not a question of whether confidentiality will be a major issue, because it always is. One of your first concerns in a new practicum setting is to find out how the facility handles client privacy issues and make sure you adhere to those procedures.

SECTION II

Professional Written Communication

4

Documentation and Technical Writing

The Basics of Writing

Good writing results in effective communication. During your day as a speech-language pathology student and professional, you may picture yourself spending most of your time talking to clients, family members, or allied professionals. While this may be the case, you will also generate various types of written communication, such as progress reports, diagnostic reports, letters, and e-mails. A well-rounded and respected clinician is competent not only in his or her interpersonal and verbal skills, but also in the content and form of his or her writing. Some professionals with whom you correspond may never have the opportunity to meet or speak with you; therefore, their impression of you rests solely on your written communication. Misspelled words, misleading or incorrect information, disorganization, tense/punctuation errors, and run-on sentences communicate to others a lack of knowledge and competence. It is vital to have the "right" information organized and written in the "right" way. In this section we get down to the nuts and bolts of professional written communication and discuss terminology and common errors students make in clinical reports.

> *Student 1:* "I'm not spending my afternoon trying to figure out how to write this when she's going to change it anyway."
>
> *Student 2:* "Yeah, I know what you mean. Mine looks like it's bleeding to death when I get it back from my supervisor—red, everywhere!"
>
> *Student 1:* "She never likes the way I say things. It's like she thinks I'm stupid or something."

Has this scenario happened to you? More than likely, if you are a student in a university SLP program, it has. What is it about reports that makes them so difficult? Why is it that information has to be written a certain way or it will be corrected? The truth of the matter is, what is written by students is not always edited/changed; it is just that documentation varies when written by different people and across work settings. The format, style, length, and degree of detail needed for a report varies across settings, university programs, and sometimes even supervisors in the same setting

(Shipley & McAfee, 2008). The differences among documentation are referenced in the appendices and throughout this book.

Some 40 years ago an article entitled, "The Agony of Report Writing: A New Look at an Old Problem" (Haynes & Hartman, 1975) addressed this. This article is still quoted extensively in dealing with professional writing (Middleton, Pannbacker, Vekovius, Sanders, & Pluett, 2001; Moon-Meyer, 2004). The reason that the article remains relevant is not that it was particularly groundbreaking or prescient, but because clinical writing still inflicts a good deal of pain on students in training, just as it always has. In that article two areas were outlined that still have the imprint of clinical relevance to students. One area was a professional terminology generator that provided examples of the kinds of terms used in clinical reports. There is a certain type of language used in professional communication, and there is no reason to keep it a secret from our students. A resource for professional terminology may include general or specific terms regarding various disorder areas. Students can use a professional terminology resource in several ways. First, when you are searching for a term to use in writing a report and you cannot think of one, you can use your textbooks or the Internet for possible examples. Second, you can use a terminology resource to reduce redundancy in reports. For example, there is redundancy in the following: "The client was stimulable for the phonemes in error. The client responded well to phonetic placement of bilabial stop consonants." Choosing another term to refer to the client would reduce redundancy in the two sentences ("The client was not stimulable for any error phonemes; however, he responded well to phonetic placement of bilabial stop consonants."). There are many ways to say that a patient "has" a particular condition (e.g., *shows*, *exhibits*, *manifests*,

demonstrates, *displays*, etc.) and you do not have to redundantly use the same term in every sentence.

There are also "professional tone words" that are often the variable that separates professional clinical communication from everyday speech. It is important to note that using discipline-specific terminology not only communicates unique information, but also maintains the integrity of our profession. We encourage you to incorporate professional terminology in your reports from the beginning and not rely on your clinical supervisor to change what you have written to increase its professional tone. The following are examples of how to use professional terminology:

- The client "produces" sounds, rather than "makes" or "says" sounds.
- The client "was observed to," rather than the clinician "saw."
- The client's performance "increased" or "improved," rather than "got better."
- "A formal test was administered," rather than "The clinician gave a test."
- "The client's performance on the test was within normal limits," rather than "The client did really well on the test."
- The client "stated" or "reported," rather than the client "said."

Tone and Language

Part of the impression you get when reading a document is related to the tone in which the writer is communicating. Tone is sometimes referred to as the "voice" or "attitude" of a piece of writing. Voice, however, may also refer to the tense you are writing in, such as passive or active. Generally, professional documents are written in the passive voice. For example, "Michael was observed to use several multiword utterances," as opposed to "Michael said four three-word sentences."

Professional tone applies to writing professional correspondence and clinical reports. If you read a letter or e-mail that appears to be immature, nonchalant, or informal, you may wonder about the professionalism of the writer. So the words you choose to use, as well as the structure of your document, will convey a specific tone, and you always want that tone to be professional. For example, you might say, "Michael has difficulty remaining on task, which may have a negative effect on his success in therapy," as opposed to "Michael won't pay attention and wiggles in his chair." The tone of each of these sentences is very different, not only because of the voice, but also because of the words that are used; "has difficulty remaining on task," sounds professional, whereas "wiggles in his chair" does not. It may be helpful to refer to a terminology resource to find appropriate professional terminology. As we alluded to earlier, it is important to have a good working knowledge of professional terminology, as you will use it frequently when writing clinical documents. It is also important, however, that information is communicated in a clear, concise manner (French & Sim, 1993). In addition, you want your communication to be appropriate for the person who will be receiving it. A letter that is being sent to a parent will not always read the same as information sent to a physician or other health care professional. Your reader should not need a dictionary, medical or otherwise, or an advanced degree to understand your letter. It has been our experience that students get so caught up in using the professional jargon they have learned that they want to "show it off." Professional terminology is not written for the purpose of impressing others with your knowledge. When communicating with other professionals, it can be a way to write detailed information in an abbreviated manner, but when communicating with parents or caregivers, it is a way to describe the results of your treatment or assessment in a way that is easy to understand. The ultimate goal is to provide the reader with clear communication of sometimes complex ideas.

Format

Using an outline each time you write will ensure the correct structure or format of your document, and generally, structure is one thing that does not change, regardless of who you are writing to or about. If you think back to when you learned to write a letter in grade school, you will recall that you were given an outline that you could use each time you sat down to write: the date in the top left or right corner, followed by the person's name and address to whom you were writing, the salutation, the body of the letter, and then, at the bottom of the page, the name of the sender. This was standard "letter writing" format, and you probably committed it to memory fairly easily. Our intention is to make the process of professional writing just as easy to learn, so that once you have mastered it, you will take that skill with you into the work setting you choose.

Common Errors

Many sources discuss common mistakes that students make when they begin writing professional reports (Haynes & Hartman, 1975; Knepflar, 1978; Meitus, 1991; Moore, 1969; Pindzola et al., 2016; Shipley

& McAfee, 2008). We feel that these frequent errors should not be kept a secret from students, but should be mentioned so that they can be proactive in clinical writing. Some of the following are errors mentioned in the above references:

1. **Redundancy:** This refers to the use of the same terms within a sentence and across abutting sentences. Redundancy can also refer to repetition of the same concept or idea. For example, the following sentences from a diagnostic report basically say the same thing: *"The results of this evaluation suggest that Joey will have little difficulty in correcting his articulation problem." "Joey's prognosis for improving his articulation skills is good."* Another example is one taken from a progress note: *"The client had difficulty remaining on task during today's session." "He was noncompliant and inattentive."*

2. **Wordiness:** Every attempt should be made to state information in the most economical way possible. Sometimes, students think that the longer a report is, the better it looks; however, reports are no place for wordy descriptions and no one wants to read more than necessary. Instead of saying, *"The client could not produce the phonemes that were in error even with multiple trials of maximum multisensory stimulation and modeling,"* it is enough to say, *"The client was not stimulable for correct production of any phonemes despite maximum cueing."* According to Strunk and White (2000), "A sentence should contain no unnecessary words, a paragraph no unnecessary sentences, for the same reason that a drawing should have no unnecessary lines and a machine no unnecessary parts" (p. 23). Good writing is concise and conveys information with efficiency. William Strunk made this perfectly clear in his famous sentence, "Omit needless words" (p. 23).

3. **Lack of professional terminology:** There are certain professional terms that are typically used in reports. Using professional terminology allows you to speak about specific skills and disorders while upholding the integrity of the profession. These terms may vary across settings but are critical to communicating a clear picture of the client's abilities. Common errors include using *"I"* instead of *"the clinician"* and using *"sounds"* for *"phonemes."* As we mention in Chapter 6, this also applies to writing treatment objectives. Making the appropriate word choice results in a well-written, measurable goal.

4. **Lack of objectivity and not separating fact from opinion:** Reports should include objective information and not unsubstantiated assumptions on the part of the clinician. Reasonable interpretation of test scores is fairly objective in terms of characterizing a client's performance in relation to standard scores. A person who scores two standard deviations below the mean could easily be considered to exhibit a disorder in the area tested. If we are talking about parent reports, we should couch these with phrases such as *"the parent reported . . . the mother stated."* If we are talking about our own opinions, this should be stated as such: *"It is the opinion of the examiner that Mary is not highly motivated for treatment."* This should be followed by a description of behaviors that support the clinician's observation such as the client's reluctance to enter the treatment room or refusal to participate in therapy activities.

5. **Lack of organization and sequence:** An organized report communicates pro-

fessionalism and is therefore more beneficial to your audience. Make sure that the appropriate information is included in the correct section of your report. For example, do not bring up history information in the clinical impressions section. A diagnostic report should be organized in such a way that it flows from background information to test results to clinical impressions and finally to recommendations. A progress note or treatment report should follow a logical sequence. The data should come before the assessment of progress and recommendations in order to paint a clear picture of what occurred during the therapy session.

6. **Ambiguity:** A sentence such as, *"The client did not perform well on the motor speech tasks,"* does not really tell us anything specific about performance. The client may not have put forth genuine effort on the task or might have demonstrated serious motoric deficits. A sentence such as, *"The client has articulation problems,"* does not tell us anything specific about the client's performance. You may not be the person in charge of the next treatment session or planning the sequence of treatment; therefore, it is important to provide the most specific details regarding performance to describe an accurate picture of the client for anyone who might read the report. A sentence such as, *"The client exhibited consistent final consonant deletion which decreased his intelligibility to 60% for unfamiliar content,"* provides the reader with a more thorough account of the client's speech and language abilities.

7. **Tense errors:** Pay attention to the nature of the section you are writing in and use the appropriate tense. You should avoid switching tenses within the same

section. Typically, the case history portion of a report or the subjective portion of a progress note is written in past tense. Later, when discussing clinical impressions and recommendations, you can switch to more active sentence constructions, because you are talking about the present and the future. *"The client's mother stated that he fell asleep in the car on the way to the clinic. She reports that he is 'grumpy.'"* A second example is *"The client produced six multiword utterances during play with blocks. He also uses single words during play activities."*

8. **Spelling and typographical errors:** In this age of spell-checkers and grammatical screeners in word processing programs, there is no excuse for spelling and typographical errors in clinical reports. Just remember that your spell-checker may not recognize clinical jargon that you have included in your report, so you may need to consult another resource such as your textbook for the correct spelling. Common spelling errors include illicit/elicit, you're/your, accept/except, and affect/effect.

9. **Wrong use of abbreviations:** It is acceptable to use an abbreviation in a report, but it should always be defined the first time it is used. A client may be administered the *Goldman-Fristoe Test of Articulation* (GFTA-4) or the *Western Aphasia Battery-Revised* (WAB-R). Once the formal title of the assessment is written, then it is okay to use the abbreviated version of the test name in later sections of the report. You may also use an abbreviation to describe a diagnosis (TBI, ADHD, CAPD, CVA), a treatment technique (LSVT, MIT, ABA), or an allied professional (OT, PT, PCP). It is important to verify that other abbreviations you choose to use are

appropriate and accepted in your facility. Appendices E and F list commonly used acronyms in medical and school settings.

10. **Use of contractions and informal language:** Reports are no place to use contracted forms (e.g., *can't, won't, we'll, he'll*, etc.). Most authorities recommend using the fully formed versions of words that are amenable to contraction. Also, the use of informal, shortened versions of words such as "*rehab*" for rehabilitation is typically not recommended. Obviously, slang terminology or colloquial terms are not acceptable in reports. Examples include "*hot mess*," "*see fit*," "*didn't get it*," "*freaked out*," and "*messed up*."

Do Not Forget Your Audience

Clinical reports end up in the hands of many different people and e-mail inboxes. It is not possible to write a report that will be equally understood by your SLP colleagues and a parent with limited educational background. Other professionals (e.g., psychologist, classroom teacher) may not understand terms that are unique to communication disorders, but if they are truly professional they will have encountered our terms before or will take the initiative to look them up. Certainly, when we receive reports from psychologists or medical doctors, they do not hesitate to use terminology unique to their fields. One solution would be to write the report to the lowest common denominator of audiences and remove all professional terms. This would help laypeople understand the report, but it would marginalize our profession. This may include those involved in the direct care of your client, such as colleagues and allied professionals, or third-party payers, which include private insurance or government-funded programs such as Medicare or Medicaid. Ultimately, your audience may be broad, and you should remember that each person has specific information in mind when reading the report. In a good clinical report, all necessary components should be included and the reader able to locate them easily. We have worked for many years to raise our profession to the same standard as other health-related professions, and part of that involves our style of reporting. One does not see psychologists, educational psychometrists, physical therapists, physicians, and occupational therapists write reports without professional language. If that were the case, a psychologist would have to explain IQ and testing methods in the report so that it would be understandable to laypersons. There are, however, schools of thought in report writing that suggest we should generate reports that are "parent friendly" or "family friendly," omitting professional terms or including definitions and explanations of concepts referred to in the report. In some ways this is good for the family, but it makes our profession seem less than it is. A family-friendly report certainly would not represent our profession as well if sent to a psychologist or physician. Discipline-specific terms exist because they allow us to refer to phenomena in an efficient and professional way. Thus, it is important for you to remember where the report is going to be sent and who is primarily going to profit from reading it. If it is going in the university clinic file, it should be written professionally for another SLP. If it is going to a public school SLP, again, it should be written professionally. If the report is going to a professional from another discipline, you should consider this while writing and define terms you feel may be unique. In medical or school settings, however, most people who work there share common terminology and freely use medical or educational terms in order to communicate most efficiently. One compromise is that some clinics write reports for the clinical file and then write a separate letter to parents summarizing the results of the evaluation in less technical terms. Other options to ensure that the results are clearly understood include sending a summary via e-mail or explaining the results over the phone or in person. There is no one way to write reports that has been agreed upon by clinics and work settings throughout the country. So, our best advice is to consider your primary audience and be as professional as possible. Ultimately, there must be a balance between communicating the pertinent information and doing so professionally. One thing is certain: You should not buy *The Big Book of Vocabulary* and learn words such as *magnanimous* or *obfuscation* and then amaze your colleagues by placing them in a clinical report.

The purpose of the present chapter has been to bring to a conscious level the notion that *any* written communication generated by the SLP puts forth an image of professionalism. The reports, letters, and e-mails that you produce reflect not only on you as a professional, but on the facility you represent. They must be organized in the correct format, written in professional language, and free of grammatical and spelling errors. Do not hesitate to take the opportunity to carefully review the documents you generate, because once you hit the "Send" button or drop that envelope in the mailbox, it is far too late for revisions.

5

Diagnostic Reports

This section begins our discussion of the formal diagnostic report. What is important to know is that the diagnostic report is sometimes the first communication someone reads about a client or patient, and therefore, it must be concise yet detailed and relevant to the patient's disorder. Miller and Groher (1990) state that the best type of report "will paint a verbal picture of a clinical case and lead the reader or listener through the collection of pertinent data to a logical diagnostic conclusion" (p. 243).

If there is one concept that is important to both professional written communication and professional verbal communication, it is *organization*. Without organization, one cannot write a coherent report, plan treatment goals/objectives, participate effectively in a multidisciplinary staffing, interview a parent, provide evaluation results, or counsel clients. Organization is one of the major variables that distinguish professional from nonprofessional communication. Thus, successful beginning students as well as veteran clinicians have one thing in common: They think a lot before they write or talk.

As indicated in the title, this chapter is concerned with diagnostic report writing, and this type of report is an excellent example of why a good clinician needs to

be organized. Think for a moment what happens in a diagnostic evaluation. Pindzola, Plexico, and Haynes (2016) illustrate that a variety of information is gathered in an evaluation. For example, you may have accumulated data in the following areas: (a) case history information, (b) prior tests and reports, (c) observation of client behavior, (d) interview findings, (e) nonstandardized testing, and (f) standardized testing. In some of these areas such as standardized testing, there may have been administration of multiple instruments. Thus, an evaluation gathers multiple sources of information, and the good diagnostician must take these disparate sources of data and synthesize them to arrive at a diagnosis. In some cases, the six sources of information may disagree. For instance, a child may pass a standardized language test but exhibit many errors in a spontaneous speech sample (nonstandardized testing). The evaluator must reconcile all of these types of information to arrive at a diagnosis. Imagine, if you will, a desk containing case history forms, notes from a parent interview, transcripts of a communication sample, prior reports from other professionals, multiple test forms, and notes from a behavioral observation, and you will see how important organization is to approaching a diagnostic report. So far, we have mentioned only the types of data you have gathered in an assessment. The diagnostic report must not only summarize all of the types of data that have been gathered, but the clinician must arrive at a diagnosis, prognosis, suggestions for further testing, clinical management suggestions, and a rationale for referral to other professionals, if appropriate. Again, as the available information is reviewed, the competent clinician is thinking about the pieces that can be used to address areas such as prognosis, treatment suggestions, and justification for referral. This requires approaching the task with an organizational structure in mind. In addition to organization, appropriate terminology is key to writing a professional diagnostic report. We illustrate some important concepts related to organization, format, and language used in diagnostic reports in the following pages. This is not meant to be a workbook for students to use in developing report-writing style. We also do not take a disorder-specific approach to reporting and provide examples from the many different disorder areas in the field. There are many sources that do a competent job of providing practice in these areas (Middleton et al., 2001; Moon-Meyer, 2004). Our intention is to talk about the variables involved in diagnostic reporting and provide some limited examples. It is important to remember that no matter how many examples are provided in a textbook, the setting in which you are working will probably do things a bit differently than the illustrations. We think that the formats, organization process, and language are the primary determinants of professional written communication, and those are what we discuss here. We also believe that it is important to illustrate diagnostic reporting as it exists across work settings at the university, medical facility, and school system.

The Organizational Framework of a Diagnostic Report

We have indicated the importance of organization to professional written communication; therefore, we discuss issues of format first. Not only is format important to organizing the writing of a report, it is also helpful in assembling all the information you have gathered during an evaluation. You can think of the sections of a report as boxes or bins in which you can place information you will later write about. One caveat before we begin: although there is always certain information that is "required" in a diagnostic report, various clinics may subdivide these evaluation summaries differently in terms of headings. There are many ways to slice and dice the information in a diagnostic report, and we present our own unique format in this text; keep in mind that we are providing an organizational framework to act as a general guide. Just remember that you will be using different headings depending on where you are working, but the information we mention will all be included somewhere in the report. Let us look at the typical sections in a diagnostic report:

- **Identifying information:** This is basic demographic information such as name, age, date of birth, case/file number, gender, address, date of the evaluation, and telephone number. It is obviously important to identify the client completely as well as when the evaluation was performed.
- **Background information:** This includes case history information from forms, prior test results, reports from other professionals, and notes from interviewing the client, family members, or parents. The importance and type of historical

information vary considerably based on the type of disorder that is present and the age of the client. For instance, neonatal, birth, and developmental history is more important for a 2-year-old than for an older child or adult. The vocational history is more important for an adult who has had a stroke than for a teenager who is still in school. Medical background is more important for clients with a medically based disorder than those with more behaviorally based problems, unless, of course, the individual has a medical diagnosis. The clinician must look at all of the case history data and interview protocols and determine which information is the most relevant to the focus of the evaluation. This section of the diagnostic report also includes the principal reason the person was referred for the evaluation. Embedded somewhere in the background information should be a statement of why the client came for services. Although this statement is not a separate section of the report, it is important to mention the client's perspective in the background information. Utilizing the "statement of the problem" will help to focus the assessment on the topic of primary concern and will determine test selection for the evaluation.

▪ **Biological bases of communication:** What we refer to in this section is auditory acuity, structure/function of the oral mechanism, and a cursory examination of neurological integrity. Most evaluations include a hearing screening to rule out auditory acuity problems or to justify referral to an audiologist for a full evaluation.

A statement of the results of the audiometric screening goes in this section and usually provides information regarding the decibel screening level and the frequencies tested. Especially in cases where motoric or structural abnormalities are suspected, we perform an oral-peripheral examination, which tests the structure and function of the oral mechanism. We also note any possible neurological symptoms such as paralysis, weakness, drooling, and deficits in fine and gross motor skill, or client reports of seizures or head injury.

This section can be quite brief if there are no remarkable findings. Obviously, the more abnormalities that are noted in structure or function of the speech mechanism, the longer this section will become.

▪ **Basic communication processes of language, articulation, voice/resonance, and fluency that are within normal limits:** When a person undergoes an evaluation for a possible communication disorder, it is assumed that the diagnostician has examined *all basic processes of communication*. For instance, we do not know that a client referred for an articulation problem does not have a language disorder as well. Thus, it is imperative that at some point in the evaluation the clinician take the time to assess, if only informally, the four areas of language, articulation, voice/resonance, and fluency. In most cases, we will not administer formal tests in the four basic areas if we can see from nonstandardized tasks such as conversation that there are no significant problems. For example, a clinician is able to determine the presence of normal vocal characteristics and fluency from listening to a conversational sample of a child that was referred for articulation errors. Especially in the university practicum setting, students might be asked to administer tests for several of the basic communication processes for the purpose of gaining experience in test administration; however, in other settings, formal testing of all areas of communication is often omitted and not reported on because they are not areas of major concern. In those cases, a clinician might not test articulation in a case that was referred for fluency, especially if no misarticulations were noted in spontaneous conversation. The bottom line here is that the diagnostic report must address, however briefly, the basic areas of communication to show that we have considered each of these as an area of possible communication disorder. This could be a brief statement such as, "With regard to age and gender, no abnormalities were noted in the client's vocal quality, resonance, articulation, or fluency."

■ **Diagnostic test results focusing on the area(s) of concern:** The bulk of the diagnostic report will involve detailing the test results on the patient's area of major concern. If that concern is a language disorder, we will be reporting the results of many standardized tests and the results of different analyses of a language sample (e.g., mean length of utterance, type-token ratio, syntactic complexity, grammatical errors, and/or pragmatic difficulties). If the concern is a fluency disorder, we will be administering and reporting many measurements of overt behaviors (e.g., frequency and type of dysfluency) and indicators of covert dimensions related to stuttering (such as feelings, attitudes, avoidances). A person whose primary concern is hoarseness will be administered many behavioral and instrumental measures of phonation during a variety of tasks ranging from prolonging vowels to connected speech. It only makes sense that the diagnostic report will devote the most space and focus to the topic of major concern.

■ **Clinical impressions and prognosis:** In this section of a report, the clinician interprets the different test results and background information to arrive at a diagnosis and prognosis. If a disorder is present, the nature and severity of the disorder should be described as well as any pertinent medical history. The prognosis for improving function should also be documented, using age, medical and communication diagnoses, family support, level of motivation, and cognitive functioning as a guide. Prognosis can be defined in terms of good, fair, poor, or guarded. This section is longer when there is disagreement among the different types of clinical data because the clinician has to explain discrepancies in results.

■ **Summary and recommendations:** This section is the most frequently read portion of a diagnostic report, especially by busy professionals. The evaluation is briefly summarized and specific recommendations for treatment, no treatment, or referral are detailed. Sometimes, the summary is included at the beginning of the report.

The organization of a diagnostic report, whether written for an adult or child client, will usually contain information from the sections presented above.

Although an evaluation done in any work setting is concerned with the same basic information we have just described, diagnostic reporting across work settings is not exactly the same. The principal difference revolves around the length of the reports. Reports in medical and school settings tend to be shorter due to (a) limitations in the use of narrative explanations and (b) report forms that limit length due to use of check boxes to indicate the presence/absence of abnormality, or a limited space allocated to note test scores. We discuss these versions of diagnostic reports in later sections.

The University Setting

Length, Content, and Format

As you probably know by now, the university clinic requires students to write detailed reports summarizing the evaluation process. In the university setting, most students begin by learning to write long narrative reports that in some cases may be five or more pages in length, depending on the type of case. It should be noted that although the report is several pages, the point is not to make the report as lengthy as possible but to be inclusive of all pertinent information that reflects the client's communication skills and your recommendations. One reason these reports are lon-

ger than in other settings is that students are often asked to administer tests that are not particularly necessary for diagnosis but are selected to give the student experience with testing. A second reason these reports are long is that students need to gain experience with professional writing. At some point in your career you might be asked to write a detailed report as part of a legal proceeding or to explain a very complicated case to another professional to whom a client is referred. In these instances, knowing how to provide clinical detail in a professional manner is important. Another reason for longer reports is that most university clinics perform comprehensive speech and language evaluations, sometimes lasting up to 2 hours. Some other settings may have evaluation time slots that extend only 20 to 30 minutes. You can simply get more testing done in 2 hours, and then you have to report the results. A final reason for the longer reports is that in the training setting, we can ask students to do more time-intensive tasks such as transcribing language samples and analyzing video recordings of play behaviors. These are important skills for students to develop. Even though such analyses represent the highest level of validity and expertise in our field, they may not be done in medical or school settings. In general, a person in a private practice, school system, or medical facility may not have the time to perform such an in-depth evaluation. However, because the university clinic is a training facility, students may be exposed to the full gamut of evaluation procedures. Thus, in the university training program you will be writing the longest of your clinical reports and you will need to learn how to pare them down in other settings. It is better, however, to know the long version before you move into more abbreviated clinical writing. As Shipley and McAfee (2008) point out, the consolation for you, the student, is that once you graduate and practice professionally, you will be able to pick and choose aspects you like from all the different models and develop your own unique style of writing.

Now we address the content of the report in a university setting. We gather so much information in a diagnostic evaluation that it is sometimes difficult to determine what is important and what is not. So, what are the ingredients of a good report? How do you get to a logical diagnostic conclusion? First, a thorough description of the patient's case history is imperative. I want to learn as much as I can about this person in the first paragraph of this report. Just as if I were reading a good book, I want something to draw me in, keep me interested, and be informative. Rambling, unimportant information is not going to keep my attention, but concise, detailed, relevant information will. Identifying information such as name, address, telephone number, and date of birth are required, and it is critical to ensure this information is correct. Sections such as background information and statement of the problem are not always straightforward, and the clinician will have to make some judgment calls on certain issues. For instance, is it more important that Jimmy likes to play soccer, or that he "can't remember anything" since he fell and hit his head on the driveway? We would vote for the head injury. It is always good to preserve the patient's or parent's statement of the problem. This is the statement that helps to guide the evaluation toward the topic of immediate concern. So, if you ask a parent why she brought her son in for an evaluation, she might say, "John has been struggling with saying his words. It's like he gets stuck and you can see the frustration on his face. I'm worried that he is beginning to stutter." That is the kind of quote that belongs in a diagnostic report because it helps to focus the evaluation and justify all of the tests and tasks you performed to assess fluency under various conditions. Speech pathology practicum students often make the mistake of not including enough pertinent information or, on the other hand, adding information that is unnecessary. A good rule of thumb is to report any information that you feel could impact speech, language, or swallowing function and describe it so that it makes sense.

Regarding other data to be mentioned in a diagnostic report, clearly the format sections we mentioned earlier will dictate the inclusion of certain types of information. Obviously, test results from standardized and nonstandardized information are important to include. After providing scores from standardized tests, it is vital to provide an explanation for what the scores reveal. After reporting test results, the diagnostic report should relate clinical impressions and prognosis, summarize the findings, and make recommendations or referrals. Usually the reporting of scores or behavioral data involves listing numerical information and perhaps some behavioral description. Clinical impressions and recommendations tend to be more narrative in nature but still based firmly on the historical information, test results, and behavioral observation.

The Medical Setting

A diagnostic report in a hospital, nursing home, or rehabilitation facility will most likely look very different from a report in the university clinic. The most noticeable differences will be the amount of information included and the format. In many medical facilities, your documentation will involve checking boxes, filling in short blanks, or writing a short description on a computer-generated form that other disciplines may be writing on as well. In some settings, you may simply record a number to represent the patient's abilities. We have included several examples of diagnostic reporting forms from a medical setting in Appendix C.

Most students who complete a practicum in a medical setting are initially thrilled when they see how "easy" these diagnostic forms are to fill out. The only drawback is you have to know exactly what information is relevant before you can accurately complete the form—this is where your practice in writing lengthy diagnostic reports comes in handy. You have already practiced figuring out what information is most pertinent and reporting it in a narrative format; now, you can apply that information to the new format. It's easy, right? Not so fast. Many of the supervisors in the medical setting whom we talked to while researching the present textbook told us that students still have difficulty "filling out the form." What we learned is that students are still tentative about which boxes to check or that they are not very familiar with the medical terminology. To help you in this area, we provide a list of the most commonly used medical terms and symbols in Appendix F.

Knowledge of terminology will be of some assistance to beginning students, but familiarity with terms alone will not alleviate your tentativeness as your pen or mouse hovers over a series of check boxes. Your greatest ally will be a logical organization of your case history data and assessment data and clear thinking about the results of the evaluation. The same procedures you went through in the university clinic are important to use in understanding the case, no matter how brief the report format. If you must choose between *aphasia* and *motor speech disorder*, you still must have thought through the evidence from your evaluation

before checking the appropriate box. The important thing is that you understand *why* you are checking a particular box on a diagnostic form.

In most cases, a diagnostic report in a hospital, nursing home, or rehabilitation facility will include the same basic information (give or take a few sections) as a diagnostic report you would write in a university clinic. Reports may still be written by hand in the chart, but will also be recorded in the facility's electronic medical record (EMR). Do not get too far ahead of yourself, though. It is still very important that you have adequate knowledge of what is important in order to be a good diagnostic reporter. As long as you use the information provided thus far, you should be on the right track.

The School Setting

Reports in the public schools vary greatly from the typical report that you would see in a medical setting, private practice, or university clinic. The information gleaned from a diagnostic evaluation may not be written down in a standard diagnostic format, as has been discussed in the previous sections, although we have seen this done in certain states. We have found that in many school systems, once the evaluation is completed, the information is compiled, discussed by the IEP team, and then transferred to an eligibility form. What you as a practicum student in the schools will see is this eligibility form. The form will include all areas of assessment, dates and names of the assessments, as well as the results. In addition, the student's strengths and needs will be included.

According to school personnel, determining strengths and needs is one of the most difficult tasks for speech pathology practicum students. Thus, the challenge of diagnostic reports in the schools is not so much in reporting the test findings, but in determining the needs of each child, based on a comprehensive evaluation.

Let's talk about what this comprehensive evaluation entails. In most public school systems, you are required to administer at least two formal assessments in language and one formal assessment in speech. The language scores will then be calculated, and, based on the standard score, it will be determined if a child is eligible for services. Eligibility determination differs by state and in some cases even by school system within the same state. Typically, a language or articulation standard score must be more than 1.5 to 2 standard deviations (SD) below the mean in order for a child to qualify for services in either speech or language disorders. Most school systems require the SLP to administer a comprehensive language assessment, one that tests both receptive and expressive language. Then, if a child shows a deficit in expressive language, for instance, the SLP must administer a formal assessment that specifically targets expressive language. According to IDEA, informal assessments can also be made part of the evaluation process. This is especially important in cases where a student may pass standardized tests but evidence errors in a spontaneous speech sample. Although informal assessments may not be considered by some school systems when determining if a child has a language delay, obtaining a language sample can be an invaluable resource in helping to "nail down" even more specific areas of deficit in children who are language impaired. Parents also have the right to seek a second opinion from a source outside the school system if they disagree with the determination of eligibility or diagnosis of their child (Haynes et al., 2006). Also, it is important to remember that there is

a significant difference between arriving at a diagnosis and determining eligibility. Diagnosis involves using standardized and nonstandardized testing to determine the existence of a communication disorder and make specific recommendations for treatment. Eligibility determination is largely an administrative operation that allows school systems to select with whom they will work. These two operations are quite different. One can have a communication disorder and may not qualify for services in the school system if it determines the disorder has no impact on educational progress or if test scores do not indicate enough of a deficit to meet criteria for eligibility.

Formal assessment is also important when evaluating a child with a fluency disorder in order to determine if the severity of the disorder warrants intervention; however, this assessment should not be limited to fluency counts, percentage of stuttered syllables, or other formal measures of severity alone. Assessment of stuttering should include discussion of the child's attitudes and emotions about his or her stuttering and consider the overall impact of the disorder on participation in the child's life (Yaruss, 2007).

At times, a child will be identified as having a voice problem during the course of a speech, language, or fluency evaluation. Because this is a subjective judgment by the speech-language clinician, it may be necessary to refer the child for medical follow-up with an ear, nose, and throat specialist (ENT). Often, the school clinician will initiate a vocal abuse awareness and/or vocal hygiene program that will be included in the child's speech goals.

Once the evaluations are finished, an eligibility form is completed. Each assessment that has been administered to the child (and the completion date) is listed, along with a description of the child's strengths and needs in each area. From there, goals are developed that target deficit areas (whether in speech, language, voice, or fluency), and benchmarks are established that will enable the SLP to help the child meet goals in the most timely and efficient manner. Figure 5–1 gives a better idea of how the diagnostic process works in the public schools.

This chapter would not be complete without a mention of computerized report writing. As you can well imagine, there are software programs for generating almost any type of document that exists. This is also true for the field of speech-language pathology. Most hospitals, private practices, and school agencies now use computer programs to generate diagnostic reports, treatment reports, progress notes, and IEPs. There are many programs available in today's market, and sometimes knowing which one to choose can be challenging. In the public schools, it has become commonplace for special educators, administrators, teachers, and SLPs to use IEP software. There are a myriad of programs available for generating IEPs, and depending on the state you are in, you may or may not be exposed to these. It is good to know about these programs and the ways that computer-generated reports may increase the efficiency of documentation of service delivery.

It is important to remember, however, that *you* are still the clinician, and the computer programs referred to above cannot think for you. This is especially critical in report writing programs that actually generate sentences based on information the clinician is prompted to provide. Always proofread the computer-generated report for accuracy and do not let the algorithms put words in your mouth, especially if they could be misinterpreted by those reading the report. No matter how a report is generated, it is always the responsibility of the clinician to ensure clarity and accuracy.

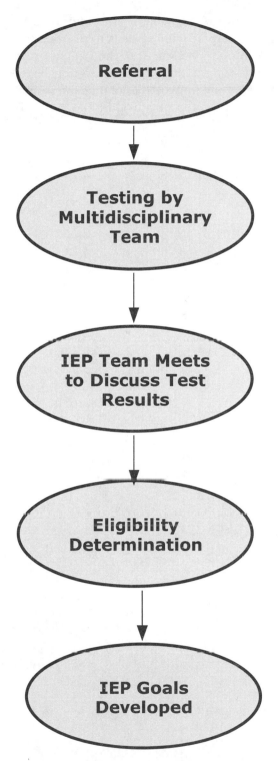

Figure 5–1. Diagnostic process in the school setting.

In closing, what is most important for you, the practicum student, to realize is that thorough assessment of the patient or client, along with a clear description of the results and implications of that assessment, is the first step in providing the most efficacious plan of care. In order to function as a competent provider of services, you must begin with an accurate, professional, and meaningful description of your patient/client's needs.

6

Treatment Documentation

Speech-language pathology is an extremely diverse and ever-changing profession that encompasses a vast array of disorders and individuals from infants to geriatrics. Clinicians are required to be exceptional problem solvers to determine the best course of treatment for each individual patient. Ongoing research, in the form of evidence-based practice (EBP), is opening doors to new avenues of treatment and new ways of understanding disorders of communication. Thus, the field of communication disorders is constantly changing. It may be daunting to you, a student, to imagine becoming competent in every area of this diverse field. However, it should be of some comfort to know that where there is change, there is also some consistency. What does *not* change is the fact that treatment of communication disorders must be planned, based on a thorough assessment, executed in a way that is efficacious and practical, and reported in a meaningful way. This chapter focuses on the process of establishing measurable goals and providing the rationales to support them. We focus on each of the various work settings and the ways in which treatment planning is similar and different for each. We also define a rationale and discuss why it is important to be able to explain why we make clinical decisions. Accurate data collection is paramount, and it is addressed as well. The reason we address these issues in a textbook on professional communication is that you will be asked repeatedly to communicate goals and rationales verbally and in many types of reports, including treatment plans and progress summaries.

In your coursework, you have no doubt dealt with the concept that thought and mental organization underlie the language we use to communicate ideas. Thus, your verbal and written communication is organized by how you think about the topic of interest. We raised this issue in the previous chapter on diagnostic reports by saying that *organization* is key to developing professional clinical writing. In the case of treatment, you must develop a principled way of thinking about goals and procedures before you can coherently talk or write about them. The process of thinking about a client's long-term goal provides you with an ultimate target you believe that client will be able to achieve in a given time period. The short-term goals are a hierarchy of steps that you follow to reach the targeted long-term goal. In psychology, this is known as successive (or progressive) approximation. We cannot expect that a client will achieve the long-term goal right away, but rather will move toward it in a systematic fashion.

In fact, the whole concept of successive approximation is based on the notion that one cannot achieve long-term goals without accomplishing short-term goals. They are the baby steps that allow a person to build competence on one level so that he or she can perform at higher levels. Clinicians must put a great deal of thought into identifying and sequencing goals of treatment so that they represent a hierarchy of difficulty leading to the ultimate long-term goal or outcome. If you have thought through the process and have a clear goal in mind, you will have much less difficulty writing a treatment plan or explaining what you are doing with a client to parents, family members, or allied professionals.

In this chapter, we discuss how to write goals and why they are an integral part of speech and language therapy reporting. We should note that our purpose in this chapter is not to provide examples of goal writing for every disorder that you might encounter in clinical practicum. Also to note is that many competent professionals may write those goals differently. Our mission is to talk about the process of goal writing and how it drives your professional communication about the client. Figure 6–1 shows the components involved in writing goals for a particular client. One component is your background knowledge gained from academic coursework. For example, you need information about normal development of the communication parameter that is affected in the client you are working with to determine the order in which typically developing individuals acquire the skill. This can be a powerful indicator of the difficulty involved in skill acquisition, and normal development is often used as a guideline in ordering treatment goals. Another aspect of background knowledge is information about the particular disorder your client exhibits. For example, if it is phonology, you should know about the types of phonological errors commonly seen in children. You should also know

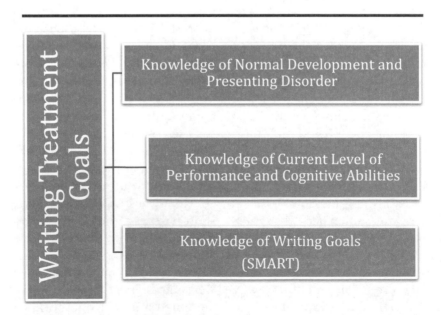

Figure 6–1. Prerequisite components of writing treatment goals.

about assessment and treatment procedures for use in treating phonological impairments. Thus, there is no substitute for background knowledge in writing goals because this information helps you to select target behaviors, sequence them in order of difficulty, and plan appropriate tasks to use in the therapy session.

A second component in writing goals is specific knowledge of your client's current level of performance and cognitive abilities. You can gain valuable information about your patient's strengths and needs from a thorough evaluation. Results from allied professionals may also impact your setting of long-term goals. For example, if a multidisciplinary evaluation revealed that your client has cognitive limitations such as an intellectual disability, a long-term goal of 100% intelligibility in sentences may not be realistic.

The third component of writing goals is the basic process of crafting observable, measurable behavioral goals. You should be able to see from Figure 6–1 that if any component is missing, the clinician will be at a loss to develop appropriate goals. It should also be apparent that a single chapter on writing goals cannot address all three components in Figure 6–1. We focus only on the mechanics of writing measurable goals in this chapter and leave it to you to combine classroom information with these guidelines. We also illustrate how these goals are similar and different in their appearance across practicum settings.

What Are Long-Term and Short-Term Goals?

After an evaluation is completed, and before beginning a program of intervention, you will have to establish the goals that you will be working toward in therapy. The essence of intervention planning is the determination of long-term intervention goals and the development of short-term goals and procedures by which to achieve them. Klein and Moses (1994) define an intervention goal as "a potential achievement by an individual with a speech-language dysfunction" that is directed toward the improvement of speech-language performance through the elimination, modification, or compensation of variables or behaviors (p. 3). The first step in planning treatment involves setting long-term goals, which will stipulate what you ultimately want your client to achieve within the specified time period. This time period will vary according to your setting and the requirements of third-party payers. Once your long-term goals are established, you can then go on to the second step, which is to prioritize target behaviors that will guide the client toward achievement of the long-term goals.

The following is an example of a long-term goal:

- The client will produce /t/ in all positions with no cuing in connected speech with 90% accuracy to increase intelligibility outside the therapeutic environment within a semester.

The following is an example of a short-term goal:

- The client will produce /t/ in the initial position of words with phonemic cues and 90% accuracy while looking at picture cards.

According to Klein and Moses (1994) a short-term goal is "a linguistic achievement that has been given priority within a hierarchy of achievements required for the realization of the long-term goal" (p. 130). In other words, the short-term goals are made up of *specific* behaviors you want to target in therapy that will enable your client to achieve long-term goals. In the previous example, the short-term goal of correct production of /t/ in words is the first step in helping the client to produce /t/ in all positions in connected speech to improve overall intelligibility. The term *given priority* means that you have chosen these behaviors to be worked on first, assuming they will result in the most effective and efficient course of treatment. Which target behaviors should be given priority? Many variables are considered, such as the severity and type of disorder, ease of teaching, natural sequence of current behaviors/prerequisite behaviors, environmental needs, and what will most significantly increase the client's function. Ultimately, it is up to you as the clinician to guide the establishment of goals; however, it is critical to involve patients and caregivers in the process. Giving the patient and caregiver a part in the planning process allows them to understand the expectations of treatment and the opportunity to provide essential input for their desired outcomes. It is worth your time to communicate with the client or caregiver to determine which goals will be most motivating and functional for the client. Functionality is of utmost importance when considering goals and implies that it will be relevant in daily life. Another phrase you may hear when discussing intervention is "quality of life," which refers to selecting goals that serve to increase the function of the person's everyday life. Both these terms indicate that you are considering the client and his or her communication needs when setting goals. You can imagine clients and their families might have increased interest in targeting a behavior in which they will see carryover into daily routines.

As the names imply, short-term and long-term goals refer to a definitive period of time. Obviously, we would not want to generate all of the possible steps leading from the client's current level of performance to the achievement of a long-term goal. That might entail scores of individual steps if you consider all of the different levels of language ranging from phoneme production to complex sentences, and all of the levels from imitative tasks to conversation. Not only would this be unwieldy, but it would not take into account the possibility of generalization and spontaneous learning on the part of the client, which might make it possible to skip planned levels of training. Thus, we limit our short-term goals to a period of several sessions. The amount of time designated for achieving a short-term goal and the number of short-term goals are often determined by where the therapy is taking place. In the university clinic, the long-term goal may be for a semester; in a hospital, it may be for a week; in a school, an academic year; and in a long-term care facility, whenever the third-party payer requires a review. Generally, in these situations, the insurance company will stipulate how long the patient is able to receive therapy. For instance, they might say 30 visits or not to exceed 8 weeks. It is, however, important to know that the procedure for choosing your short-term goals is virtually the same across work settings and various lengths of treatment. The bottom line is that you need to think about how many short-term steps the client can realistically accomplish in the time frame allotted (semester, school year, 2 weeks in a rehabilitation facility, or a week in acute care).

An important issue to consider is that most often a client will have more than a single short-term goal. Short-term goals often interlock with one another, and they represent different facets of the same underlying aspect of client growth. For example, a child who has a limited expressive lexicon of 40 words at age 3 might have a short-term goal (STG) of increasing lexicon size to 75 words. This client might also have a STG of increasing mean length of utterance (MLU) from 1 to 2. To increase this MLU, specific types of word combinations might be targeted such as basic operations of reference (more + X, that + X, allgone + X) and two-term semantic relations (agent + action; action + object). Thus, this child has several STGs that involve increasing expressive lexicon size, increasing MLU, increasing use of basic operations of reference, and increasing use of certain two-term semantic relations. When you think about it, all four STGs relate to teaching the child to use multiword utterances. All of this could potentially be accomplished in a university setting during the course of one semester. Pertinent factors in determining how many short-term goals to target for each given period of time include the client's age and cognitive ability, current level of functioning, severity and type of the disorder, behavior, frequency and duration of therapy, and participation and compliance with a home program.

What Is a Goal?

A goal is a statement that describes the intended target behavior in an observable and measurable way. The goal is the staple of everyday treatment planning. Think of the goal as an instruction manual or a blueprint for how to conduct a therapy session. Just as with building a house, it is difficult to get started without the blueprint. Similarly, without the instruction manual, you would not know how to put together a bookcase, for example, or a child's swing set. You must have a plan for how to conduct a therapy

session, and your goals are your plan. Those goals dictate not only your behavior in the treatment session but also how you talk and write about what you do in professional communication.

The first thing to remember about goals is they must be something you can both observe and measure. In order to accomplish this, the clinician must identify what the client is expected to do, under what conditions, and with what degree of success. Owens, Metz, and Farinella (2011, p. 96) suggest that the letters ABCD are helpful in remembering the format for writing behavioral goals:

A. Audience: Who is expected to demonstrate the behavior?
B. Behavior: What is the observable and measurable behavior?
C. Condition: What is the context or condition of the behavior?
D. Degree: What is the targeted degree of success?

With this "blueprint" you should be able to write a measurable goal for any behavior that you wish to target in therapy.

Example 1:

A. Betty
B. will produce /s/
C. in the initial position of words while naming pictures with no cues
D. with 90% accuracy after three consecutive sessions.

Example 2:

A. Karen
B. will include narrative elements of setting and character
C. in a story in response to sequence pictures with a choice cue
D. in three out of five opportunities after four therapy sessions.

Example 3:

A. Amanda
B. will increase the number of words to request or label
C. during 15 minutes of structured play with the clinician with no cues
D. to a minimum of 20 single words after six sessions.

Example 4:

A. James
B. will utilize smooth, controlled speech
C. with an unfamiliar listener inside the therapy room during a 5-minute conversation
D. in 50% of communicative opportunities after two therapy sessions.

As long as you have identified your client's deficits, based on a thorough assessment, you should be able to apply this formula to create appropriate goals for treatment. Note that in the above examples we have specified the stimulus or condition, the task, and the target response. Degree may be measured in time, number, or frequency. Time periods are frequently referred to by the number of sessions but can also be referenced in terms of specific dates. These are critical components to include in long- and short-term goals.

Another way of conceptualizing the abstract art of goal writing was defined by Neal (2005) and includes thinking through the following questions after determining what skills you want to develop. The guiding questions are as follows: Who?, Will do what?, How well?, and Under what conditions? So, for example, Who? (Julie); Will do what? (suppress the phonological process of fronting in words); How well? (with 80% accuracy after four therapy sessions); Under what conditions? (following the clinician's model during structured play).

An additional consideration for goal writing is to assess once you have written your goal, if it is "SMART." This is an acronym for ensuring that your goal is Specific, Measurable, Attainable, Relevant, and Timely. Torres (2013) outlines guidelines for making sure your goals are "smart." Let's look briefly at each of these in Table 6–1.

In order to write measurable goals, it is wise to consider what words you may and may not want to use.

Table 6–1. SMART Goals

Specific	This involves assessing the skills your client needs to develop, their current abilities, and tasks that will target these skills.
Measurable	The skill you are targeting must be clear and performance able to be assessed.
Attainable	Is the goal something the client can be expected to achieve in a reasonable time frame?
Relevant	Does the goal serve to increase the client's social or academic needs? Will it increase their ability to communicate?
Timely	The goal should include a time frame and it should indicate a time period that is feasible for the client to attain the goal.

Selected words to *avoid* in writing goals:

Understand, listen, enjoy, think, know, review, develop an appreciation, like, comprehend, feel, learn, become able, attain, grasp, memorize, acquire, discover, discern, assimilate, digest, grasp, perceive, recognize

We suggest avoiding such words because they are *not measurable and observable*. It is critical for clinicians, patients, caregivers, and third-party payers to be able to track progress, and progress can only be monitored if the goal is measurable and observable.

Selected words that may be useful in writing behavioral goals:

Define, describe, identify, label, list, match, name, outline, select, state, explain, give example, paraphrase, summarize, compute, predict, produce, show, solve, use, diagram, differentiate, discriminate, distinguish, recall, illustrate, outline, select, categorize, compose, organize, plan, rewrite, write, tell, compare, contrast, justify, interpret, ask, choose, follow directions, give, locate, point to, sit, reply, take turns, answer, comply, greet, perform, read, initiate, share, work, combine

What Is a Rationale?

One of the most important questions you can ever ask yourself, in any situation, is, "Why do I do what I do?" This is certainly true in the field of SLP with intervention planning. Establishing a rationale for your treatment protocol is extremely important, possibly one of the most important aspects

of your training. So, that being said, let's talk about rationales and how they are used in therapy.

Merriam-Webster's Dictionary defines *rationale* as "the reason or explanation for something." If you look up the word *rationale* in a thesaurus, you will see words such as *justification*, *basis*, and *reasoning*. As this applies to speech-language treatment, you must have a basis, or reasoning, for what you do with your clients. The rationale for your treatment should be based upon evidence-based practice. In 2004, ASHA's executive board stated that the goal of EBP is the integration of (a) clinical expertise/expert opinion, (b) external scientific evidence, and (c) client/patient/caregiver perspectives "to provide high-quality services reflecting the interests, values, needs, and choices of the individuals we serve." Dollaghan (2004, p. 3) identifies EBP as "a framework and a set of tools" that allows us to "upgrade our knowledge base" to be better clinicians.

When you use EBP to determine your course of action with a client, you will be able to structure therapy goals with the latest research and your previous experiences, and also with the client's individual needs at the forefront. In essence, all of the therapy techniques that are being used today, regardless of the specific area (voice, fluency, articulation, language, swallowing, etc.), are used because there is at least some research evidence that shows these techniques are effective. In cases where research evidence is lacking, we should at least be able to provide a theoretical justification for what we decide to do in treatment. This is where the two components of your graduate program, academic and clinical, come together. In your academic training, you will gain the foundational knowledge of each disorder, which includes, but is not limited to, theoretical bases for communication disorders, assessment protocols, and various treatment techniques. You will also become familiar with the research that supports it. Once you have knowledge of the nature of disorders and assessment/treatment techniques that have been proven effective by research, you can begin to apply it to your clinical preparation (Figure 6–2). Regardless of the setting to which you are assigned for practicum, it makes sense that you would use EBP when formulating goals. If you have considered your rationale for each goal and activity, you will be ready to explain why you are choosing to work on certain targets. You want to be ready with your answer when your client, their caregivers, or colleagues inquire about aspects of your treatment plan.

What Is Data?

You can have the perfect session planned with regard to activities and reinforcement, but if you do not take the time to collect data, you have missed the boat. Although you may perceive that your client's articulation is better, data collected during your session can substantiate your opinion. When communicating with the client, his or her family, and other professionals, your data will be the goal foundation on which you base your recommendations. Not only should you gather data during each trial of the target behavior, but you want to ensure that your data are accurate. Accurate data collection is essential in providing meaningful and effective services to your clients. Olswang and Bain (1994, p. 58) stress the importance of data in making accurate clinical decisions and note that data collection involves three preliminary steps, including making the decision of what to measure, how to measure, and how frequently to measure. Careful thought should be given to these steps, in that reliable and valid data should answer questions including what is effective in therapy, what needs to be modified, and when your client is meeting his or her goals.

Olswang and Bain (1994, p. 57) identify three principles that are paramount for data

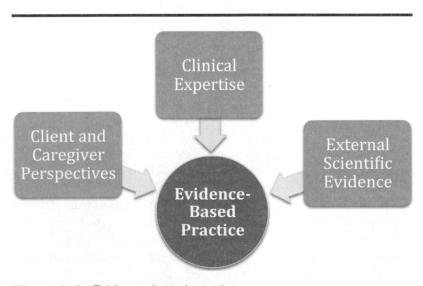

Figure 6–2. Evidence-based practice.

and methods of collection. These include that the data must be valid, reliable, and "collected in a reasonable fashion." As long as you are collecting data in a consistent manner, you may format your data sheet in any way you would like. Depending on the client's disorder and target behaviors, you may have a different format for each client. When deciding how to structure your session, it will be helpful to think about what target behavior you are taking data on, the cues, and the criteria. You should make every effort to take data during the session; however, the target behavior or individual client needs may preclude this. We have included several examples of data sheets in Appendix H for your reference. Data are usually reported in your progress note or other places as dictated by the setting you are in at the time. However, your data sheet may or may not be included in the client record. Regardless, baseline data should be obtained the first time the goal is targeted to have a way to measure progress. Calculating progress or lack thereof toward goals guides your decision of when to modify goals and cues to best serve your client and his or her level of functioning. A helpful tool in tracking progress is a long-term graph. Long-term graphs make it easy to quickly determine if and when a goal is met. Please refer to Appendix J for examples.

In addition, the implementation of cues or prompts should be documented. A cue is something provided by the clinician to help the client achieve the target behavior when he or she is not capable of producing it independently. There are many different types of cues including verbal cues, full model cues, and tactile cues. Your initial decision of which types of cues to use varies according to the client's disorder and level of functioning. Analysis of the effectiveness of the cues as represented in data collection may lead to your cuing hierarchy

being altered. Based on your client's level of ability, cuing may be incorporated into your goal or your goal may be for the client to achieve the target without cues or independently.

Maintaining consistent and accurate data is paramount to determining when to discharge clients and offering support for your recommendations. Hegde and Davis (2010, p. 290) consider a target behavior to be trained "when its production in conversational speech in natural settings is acceptable." For example, Hegde and Davis (2010) recommend the following criteria:

- "minimum of 90% accuracy for phonemes and language structures in conversational speech"
- "at least 90 to 95% of utterances or of speaking time for normal voice characteristics"
- disfluencies not to exceed 3 to 4% in conversation outside the therapy environment

Although these guidelines may be appropriate for most clients, your competence as a growing clinician may lead you to discharge your client prior to reaching this criterion.

All settings, no matter how disparate they might appear at first glance, require practitioners to state goals and goals, and these statements are always in written form. The following sections are designed to illustrate how goals and goals are similar yet slightly different across work/practicum settings.

The University Setting

Most of you will begin your practicum experience in a university clinic. It is for this reason that throughout this book, we include examples of what forms and reports might look like in this setting. In the university setting, your paperwork requirements are most likely more involved than in any other practicum environment. As we said in an earlier chapter, the intensity of the university setting in requiring rationales, goals, procedures, and detailed reports is a valuable learning experience. As a beginning clinician in the university clinic, you may be asked to write a rationale for each goal you develop, and even though you will not continue to do this, it is good practice when you are gaining experience and confidence in goal writing. It teaches you how to think about clinical work and enables you to explain your approaches in any amount of detail required. If you gain experience writing behavioral goals from scratch in the university clinic, you will have a lot less trouble selecting the check boxes on an electronic form in a medical setting or using a goal bank in a school system. Again, what is important is the thought process and understanding *why* you choose to work on certain goals as a pathway to helping your client.

With the guidance of clinical supervisors, you will find that the university clinic is an excellent setting in which you can learn the "ins and outs" of becoming a competent speech-language clinician. Because a university clinic traditionally operates on a semester-by-semester basis, your long-term and short-term goals are influenced by this time frame. We now examine what long-term and short-term goals might look like in the university clinic.

The Integration of Long-Term Goals (LTGs), Short-Term Goals (STGs), and Rationales

Because you will see a number of different disorders across the life span in the university clinic, goals may be written many different ways. As mentioned previously, using the ABCD formula may be helpful when writing goals, even when the goal is written in a simple sentence. Below are examples of long-term goals with a short-term goal (STG) and a rationale for each goal.

Client 1: 3-year-old male

Diagnosis: Limited expressive lexicon, normal receptive vocabulary, only uses single-word utterances (MLU 1.0).

LTG 1: The client will verbally express wants and needs with minimal cueing in all contexts with familiar and unfamiliar listeners and 75% accuracy by the end of the semester.

STG 1: (A) The client (B) will increase his expressive lexicon size to 75 (C) in naming tasks with verbal cues (D) at home and in clinical sessions as measured by sampling and parent reporting on a lexicon checklist across a week's time.

Rationale: Two-word utterances are typically not produced by normally developing children until the lexicon size exceeds 50 (Nelson, 1973).

STG 2: (A) The client (B) will increase MLU to 2.0 (C) during play (D) after 2 weeks at home and in the university clinical setting.

Rationale: Brown's stages of language development (Brown, 1973) indicate that a 3-year-old child should have a MLU of 2.5 to 3.9.

STG 3: (A) The client (B) will increase production of the basic operations of reference (nomination + X, recurrence + X, and nonexistence + X), (C) in structured play, (D) after a 3-week interval at home, and in the university clinical setting.

Rationale: Brown (1973) reported that the first types of word combinations seen in normal development are the basic operations of reference.

STG 4: (A) The client (B) will increase the production of the two-term semantic relations of agent + action and action + object, (C) during play following a verbal prompt (D) after six therapy sessions.

Rationale: Brown (1973) reported that agent + action and action + object are early developing semantic relations and they are the basis for SVO constructions.

Client 2: 22-year-old female

Diagnosis: Bilateral vocal nodules

LTG 1: The client will improve voice quality to 80% accuracy in conversation without cuing within five sessions using a Resonant Voice technique.

STG: (A) The client (B) will smooth voice quality using Resonant Voice technique (C) in structured tasks with auditory and kinesthetic cuing (D) to 80% accuracy after three therapy sessions.

Rationale: Anterior or forward focus of the voice results in less abuse of the vocal folds and improved resonance (Boone, McFarlane, Von Berg, & Zraick, 2014).

Client 3: 5-year-old female

Diagnosis: Articulation disorder

LTG 1: The client will produce /k/ and /g/ in all positions at the phrase level with no cues during structured tasks

with 90% accuracy after 12 therapy sessions.

STG 1: The client will produce /k/ initial in words following the clinician's model with a visual stimulus with 90% accuracy within four sessions.

Rationale: According to Smit et al. (1990), 90% of females have acquired /k/ by the time they are 3 years, 6 months old; /k/ is an early developing phoneme.

Client 4: 22-year-old male

Diagnosis: Fluency disorder

LTG 1: The client will utilize appropriate fluency shaping techniques and strategies with no cues to increase verbal fluency in academic and social settings with 80% accuracy within eight sessions.

STG 1: The client will use Easy Onset while reading three- to four-word phrases with verbal cues in 8 out of 10 trials after three therapy sessions.

Rationale: Many people who stutter have difficulty on the initial word in an utterance; the Easy Onset or Easy Relaxed Approach (ERA) technique has proven very effective in initiating speech (Gregory, 2002).

Client 5: 33-year-old male

Diagnosis: English as a second language (ESL); difficulty with pronunciation of English phonemes.

LTG 1: The client will use Standard American English (SAE) with 70% accuracy during conversation with unfamiliar listeners with minimal cues in order to communicate more effectively in vocational and social settings after 10 sessions.

STG 1: The client will discriminate between minimal pairs /b/ and /v/ in words when provided with auditory stimuli on the first attempt for 90% accuracy.

STG 2: The client will produce /v/ initial in words while reading from a word list with no cuing and 90% accuracy across five sessions.

Rationale: Van Riper and Emerick (1995) recommend that discrimination training occur prior to production training during the establishment phase of treatment; in addition, Locke (1980) states that only error sounds should be included in speech sound discrimination training.

Appendix D shows an example of a university clinic treatment plan.

The Medical Setting

Setting goals in medical facilities is somewhat different from that in the university clinic, mainly due to the time frame of therapy and health care requirements. Any patient who receives speech therapy services in a medical facility will more than likely be covered by an insurance plan or plans (if he has private insurance in addition to Medicare or Medicaid). Entities that pay a portion or the entire fee for services on an individual's behalf are often referred to as third-party payers.

All health care facilities in the United States are governed by federal laws that regulate how payments are made, the codes used for billing, and the amount of time a patient can receive services. The Centers for Medicare and Medicaid Services (CMS) have the most updated information on Medicare billing procedures and regulations. You can find them on the Internet (http://www.cms.hhs.gov).

When requesting payment from a third-party payer for speech therapy services, the speech-language pathologist has to enter a billing code that corresponds with the patient's diagnosis and/or treatment. Diagnosis codes are published by the World Health Organization and are known as ICD-10 codes. This stands for *International Classification of Diseases, Tenth Revision, Clinical Modification*. You will most likely hear them referred to as ICD-10 codes. Billing codes for treatment, also known as CPT or *Current Procedural Terminology* codes, are published by the American Medical Association and are used in conjunction with ICD-10 codes. CPT codes, originally intended for physicians, are now used widely by many other practitioners (e.g., SLP, physical therapy, occupational therapy). All clinical documentation in a medical facility must support the codes that are billed. This also determines to some extent how goals are written and executed in a medical setting.

As is the case in the university clinic, the SLP will first decide on a long-term goal for a patient in a medical facility; however, this is not true for all medical facilities. Some hospitals do not establish long-term goals, simply because a short-term goal is more efficacious. A hospital patient may be in an acute care unit for just a few days. In this case, a long-term goal is not necessary. For rehabilitation hospitals, the patient may only remain in a rehabilitation hospital for 7 to 21 days so long-term goals are written accordingly.

In writing a long-term goal for a patient in any type of medical facility, several factors must be taken into consideration. The SLP usually writes a long-term goal as a first step in establishing a *plan of care* (POC); however, there must be a written order from a physician requesting an evaluation and treatment for speech. For Medicare patients, the plan of care must not only be established and certified by a physician before treatment begins, it must be recertified by the physician after a certain time period has elapsed.

In the following section, we provide examples of long-term goals as they would be written in a rehabilitation facility, hospital, and extended care setting. Keep in mind that in most medical facilities, there is often a "menu" of long-term goals listed, and the SLP will simply check the appropriate goal; however, as a clinical practicum student, you will be expected to discern which goals will be appropriate for your patients based on the evaluation report.

You should know that *functional* is the operative word when writing speech and language goals for any patient, but especially so in the medical setting. To that end, *activities of daily living* (ADLs) are often mentioned in patient goals. Activities of daily living include activities such as bathing, grooming, cooking, housekeeping, and personal hygiene.

The Rehabilitation Setting

In this setting, patients are typically admitted from an acute care facility to increase their level of function and independence before going home. Documentation is most likely completed on a computer, and general goals are provided as guidelines. Of course, each goal is individualized for the patient to tailor to his or her needs. Documentation revolves around functional levels and FIM scores. *Functional independence measures*, or FIM scores, which are widely

used in rehabilitation settings, are listed below. These were developed by the Uniform Data System for Medical Rehabilitation at the State University of New York at Buffalo. It is assumed that a patient who needs moderate assistance will be targeting the next higher level of independence (minimal assistance) as therapy progresses. At this point it is useful to provide a brief summary of FIM scores that you might see in medical treatment goals. The FIMs are used in medical facilities to gauge admission and discharge status of the patient and document progress in a variety of areas. In this setting, SLPs are usually responsible for assigning FIM scores to the following areas: comprehension, expression, memory, attention, problem solving, swallowing, and social interaction. Other disciplines such as nursing, physical therapy, and occupational therapy have their respective areas to score but may score these same areas as well. Additional areas rated by team members include bowel/bladder, stairs, eating, grooming, and bathing.

7—Complete independence (timely, safely)

6—Modified independence (extra time, devices)

5—Supervision (cuing, setup)

4—Minimal assist (performs 75% or more of task)

3—Moderate assist (performs 50% to 74% of task)

2—Maximal assist (performs 25% to 49% of task)

1—Total assist (performs less than 25% of task)

Accurate FIM scores are vital as they guide the decision of the third-party payer as to how many days the patient may remain at the rehabilitation facility. They also provide an indicator of the level of assistance, if any, the patient will need when they are discharged. Below you will find a sampling of some long-term goals from a rehabilitation facility. We also provide several examples of one short-term goal that might accompany these long-term goals. In addition to the following, a level of assistance may be specified after the goal.

Sample Long-Term Goals

At first glance, these goals may seem confusing or like a foreign language. Once you see them every day, however, they will begin to make sense and soon will become a regular part of your vocabulary.

- Patient will answer verbally presented questions at the word level with 70% accuracy with no cues to increase understanding of therapy instructions/conversation.
- Patient will use dysarthria compensatory strategies in single-syllable words with 80% accuracy with tactile cues with familiar listeners to increase intelligibility of verbal communication.
- Patient will use an external memory aid with 60% accuracy with gestural cues to maximize memory skills.
- Patient will express abstract information using an augmentative system with 90% accuracy with verbal cues to increase functional communication.
- Patient will perform money management tasks with 75% accuracy with written cues to increase independence with home management/community functioning.

- Patient will point to actions with 90% accuracy to increase comprehension and communication for basic wants/needs.
- Patient will use compensatory safe swallowing strategies with a mechanical soft diet and nectar-thick liquids with 80% accuracy with no cues to decrease risk of aspiration.

As is evident from this list of goals, one of the most important factors in establishing long-term goals for patients in a medical facility is that the patient will be able to resume, to the greatest degree possible, his or her premorbid lifestyle. If written in the patient's chart, the goal may be written in an abbreviated form [e.g., $\uparrow$ verbal expression and problem solving from MAX (2) to MOD (3),] with the "up arrow" meaning increase or improve. In the following examples, FIM scores are in parentheses after the corresponding level of assistance required.

LTG: Patient will express basic wants and needs through single words with a familiar listener with 77% accuracy and verbal cues.

STG: Patient will increase ($\uparrow$) verbal expression for common object identification from MOD (3) to MIN (4).

LTG: Patient will use functional problem solving with 50% accuracy with verbal cues to increase safety during ADL tasks.

STG: Pt will $\uparrow$ verbal reasoning and problem solving from Total (1) to MAX (2).

LTG: Patient will follow simple one-step commands with 90% accuracy to increase comprehension for community tasks.

STG: Pt. will ↑ comprehension for simple one-step commands from MOD (3) to MIN (4).

LTG: Patient will produce phrases with 70% accuracy with visual cues to develop voluntary control over apraxic symptoms.

STG: Pt. will ↑ intelligibility at phrase level from MAX (2) to MOD (3).

LTG: Patient will read and comprehend newspapers with 70% accuracy with no cues to increase functional reading comprehension.

STG: Pt. will ↑ reading comprehension at the phrase level from MAX (2) to MOD (3).

LTG: Patient will independently utilize strategies to increase safety while eating a regular consistency diet with thin liquids.

STG: Pt. will ↑ completion of OMEs from MIN (4) to SPV (5).

LTG: Patient will answer yes/no questions related to personal information with verbal cues to increase effectiveness of comprehension within the environment.

STG: Pt. will ↑ reliability for answering simple yes/no questions from MAX (2) to MOD (3).

LTG: Patient will write phrases with verbal cues using the dominant hand to increase functional writing for ADLs.

STG: Pt. will ↑ written expression for content of checks from MAX-2 to MOD-3.

The Hospital Setting

As mentioned previously, the SLP in an acute care setting, such as in a hospital, may not develop long-term goals for patients, simply because the duration of their stay does not warrant them. In this case, the SLP will write one or more short-term goals for the patient, based on the initial evaluation. There will more than likely be a description of the patient's deficits included in the evaluation report, and it will be the job of the SLP to develop short-term goals based on this information. The short-term goals will be similar to the ones listed above or may also be chosen from a menu of goals on a computer on a preprinted form. Often, abbreviations will be used instead of words. Refer to Appendix F for a partial list of common medical abbreviations, but keep in mind that these abbreviations may vary by state and facility. Below is an example of short-term goals for patients in a hospital setting:

Patient 1: 72-year-old male

Primary diagnosis: Aphasia

STG 1: Increase (↑) auditory comprehension of one-step commands to 80% accuracy.

STG 2: Increase auditory comprehension of simple yes/no questions to 80% accuracy.

STG 3: Increase automatic speech to 80% accuracy.

STG 4: Increase ability to name objects to 75% accuracy.

Patient 2: 36-year-old male

Primary diagnosis: TBI

STG 1: Oriented to time, place, and situation with visual cues with 90% accuracy.

STG 2: Provide biographical information verbally when prompted with 80% accuracy.

STG 3: State solution to verbal, functional problem-solving situations related to ADLs with 75% and moderate assistance.

Patient 3: 80-year-old female

Primary diagnosis: Dysarthria

STG 1: Pt will demonstrate adequate breath support and coordinate breathing and phonation while reading single words from a list independently in 8 out of 10 trials.

STG 2: Increase speech intelligibility at the single-word level to 70% accuracy.

Note that abbreviations are often used in a hospital setting, as well. In these examples, OME stands for *oral motor exercises* and an up arrow indicates "improve" or "increase." Patients usually do not remain in an acute care setting for an extended period of time, and your goal, if you are the SLP who is treating this patient, is to figure out what will be most beneficial to this patient during his stay in acute care. This is based on information collected during the patient's evaluation, concomitant medical conditions, input from the family (when available), and the patient's prognosis.

Long-Term Care/Skilled Nursing Facility

Long-term care (LTC), *extended care, skilled nursing facility* (frequently referred to as SNF), and *nursing home* are names that apply to a facility that provides a range of health, personal care, social, and housing services to people who are unable to care for themselves independently. The SLP who works in one of these facilities will perform many of the same services as an SLP in a hospital or rehabilitation setting; the main difference is the duration of services provided, and this is determined in large part by Medicare.

Any student who has a practicum experience in a LTC facility will become familiar with Medicare, and the terms *Part A* and *Part B*. For the purpose defined in this text, you will not need to have a detailed knowledge of Medicare and its components; however, it is important to know that patients are billed either under Part A or Part B, depending on their age, diagnosis, and length of stay in the facility. Patients who are considered *acute* and are receiving skilled nursing, usually in the first 100 days following their move from the hospital to the LTC facility, are billed under Part A. Patients who are considered more *chronic* and have been in the LTC facility for more than 100 days are billed under Part B (i.e., a patient suddenly begins having difficulty swallowing and is referred to the SLP for evaluation and treatment, even though he has been in the LTC facility for 8 months).

Another reason we mention Part A and Part B in this section is that the requirement for progress notes is different for each one: for Part A, the SLP will complete a weekly note, and for Part B he will complete a daily note. Because most patients in a LTC facility are covered by Medicare, this billing system is the driving force behind how therapy is carried out as well as how all of the supporting paperwork is completed.

Let's examine what goals may look like in a long-term care or nursing home setting. Some LTC facilities provide a "goal bank" for long-term and short-term goals. The following are some examples of long-term goals.

Long-term goals may include

- The patient will recall personal information with the use of compensatory strategies to improve carryover from day to day, and to improve safety.
- The patient will facilitate safe swallowing skills with the least restrictive diet via use of compensatory strategies, diet modifications, and caregiver/family education with 90% accuracy.
- The patient will improve expressive language skills for complex conversations in order to increase communication competence in a SNF setting.
- The patient will tolerate highest possible diet with the use of compensatory strategies 100% of the time without signs/symptoms of aspiration to optimize nutrition and hydration.
- The patient will improve cognitive function including attention skills to independent, memory skills to supervision and problem-solving abilities to supervision to allow for increase functional integration into environment and complete activities of daily living.
- The patient will focus attention to tasks for 10 minutes with 80% accuracy with verbal instruction/cues for therapy tasks.

Short-term goals may include

- The patient will name objects, pictures, people, and/or activities independently in order to improve verbalizations.
- The patient will perform verbal sentence completion tasks increasing

to minimal level of impairment given 5% verbal instruction/cues to increase automatic verbalizations.
- The patient will communicate/verbalize mental awareness of person, place, and time (×3) given 50% verbal instruction/cues in order to increase functional integration into environment.
- The patient will improve safety awareness for self-care tasks with minimal assistance (1%–25% assist).
- The patient will perform two-step daily living tasks given 25% visual and verbal instruction/cues, increasing to mild impairment level in order to increase independence with daily routine.
- The patient will execute oral-motor exercises with 85% no instruction/cues upon visual model for increased control and movement of bolus to minimize the risk of aspiration.

Although goals in a LTC setting may not always be written in this way, two things are usually true regarding goals for patients in a medical setting: (a) they are meant to be functional and (b) they are written in order to restore the patient, to the greatest extent possible, to his or her prior level of functioning.

The School Setting

Any student who completes a speech pathology clinical practicum in the public schools will encounter the *Individualized Education Program*, or IEP. For any students who have an opportunity to serve children ages birth to 3 years, whether in a preschool, Head Start, or Early Intervention program, the *Individualized Family Services Plan*, or IFSP, will also become familiar. In order for you to understand treatment planning and goal setting in the public school environment, we need to provide some background. It is important for you to know that school systems operate the way they do not because of arbitrary decisions made by school districts, but due to the existence of many complex layers of federal and state law.

Individualized Education Program (IEP)

The IEP is a written plan outlining the special education program and/or other services (speech therapy) required by a particular student. It identifies learning expectations that are modified from or alternative to the expectations for the appropriate grade and subject, including measurable goals and benchmarks for each goal. It also identifies any accommodations or modifications needed to assist the student in achieving his or her learning expectations. In addition, the IEP provides a framework for monitoring and reporting progress to parents.

Every student who has been identified as eligible for special education services of any kind must have an IEP. This applies to students who receive speech therapy as a part of other special education services, as well as to students who are served through the general education curriculum and are "pulled out" for speech therapy.

To create an effective IEP, parents, teachers, administrators, other related services personnel, and sometimes even the student must come together to determine unique needs. These individuals must design an educational program that will help the student be involved in the general curriculum to the greatest extent possible and make educational progress.

The Individuals with Disabilities Education Act (IDEA) requires certain information to be included in each child's IEP; however, states and local school systems often include additional information in IEPs in order to meet federal or state laws. The flexibility that states and school systems have to design their own IEP forms is one reason why IEP forms may look different across school systems or states (United States Department of Education [DOE], 2000).

No Child Left Behind (NCLB) was passed on January 8, 2002, and also impacted the operation of school systems. NCLB was built on four principles: (a) accountability for results, (b) more choices for parents, (c) greater local control and flexibility, and (d) an emphasis on doing what works based on scientific research. We do not entertain a detailed discussion regarding NCLB in this book, and it should be noted that many states have now moved away from NCLB due to recent changes in the law.

The IEP Development Process

As mentioned previously, the IEP is a written description of a specific instructional program for a student with special needs. In order to understand IEP goals, it is useful to know how an IEP is generated. The IEP is developed by a multidisciplinary team of professionals, so the SLP is not writing goals in a vacuum. There are six steps that must be followed in the process of establishing an IEP for any student:

1. **Pre-referral:** This is an informal process that involves the classroom teacher identifying the student's educational problems and suggesting solutions. These interventions are attempted for a 6-week period. In some states, this is part of the Response to Intervention (RTI), which is a three-tiered approach

designed to minimize the number of children who are referred for special education services. RTI is composed of the following:

a. Tier 1: Core Instruction
b. Tier 2: Group Intervention
c. Tier 3: Intensive Intervention

More information on RTI may be found at http://www.rtinetwork.org

2. **Referral:** If the interventions put in place during the pre-referral are not successful, then a referral for an evaluation is made. A verbal or written request can be made by the child's parent or teacher. It should be noted that only those students with academic performance extensively behind that of their classmates and/or those who exhibit learning, emotional, and behavioral difficulties can be officially referred. Once the referral is made, an IEP team is created. This team consists of the student's parent(s)/guardian, special education teacher, one general education teacher, and any other professionals who may need to provide services to the student.

3. **Evaluation:** Once the referral has been made, the student must be evaluated to determine if a disability exists, whether special education is required, and, if so, what types of special or related services are needed. The type of evaluation that is performed will be based on the deficits identified during the pre-referral and referral processes. Tests may be administered to assess learning, communication, behavior, or a combination of modalities. Federal law mandates that the IEP team must administer at least two formal assessments in the student's native language in order to determine eligibility for special education. The team has 60 days from the referral date to determine eligibility.

4. **Eligibility:** Once the results of the evaluation are prepared, the IEP team will meet to determine if the student meets eligibility requirements. To be eligible, the child must meet the criteria defined by IDEA as a "child with a disability." There must be a unanimous decision by the team for the student to be referred for special education services.

5. **Development of an IEP:** Within 30 days of the eligibility determination, the team will decide on the appropriate services and placement for the student, preferably in the least restrictive environment (LRE). A broad definition of LRE is an educational setting where a child with disabilities can receive a free appropriate education designed to meet his or her needs while being educated with peers without disabilities in the regular education environment to the maximum extent appropriate. It is during this phase of IEP development that specific goals are generated. We discuss this specifically in the next section.

6. **Service provision:** The child's teachers and caregivers should have copies of the IEP and be familiar with his or her specific responsibilities. Accommodations, modifications, and supports are all included in the IEP. Progress toward annual goals is frequently measured and the child's parents are informed of performance on a consistent basis.

7. **Annual review:** The IEP team is responsible for conducting an annual review to ensure that the student is meeting goals and/or making progress on the benchmarks specified for each goal that was developed by the team. This review takes place on a yearly basis; however, if the IEP needs to be modified or otherwise updated, a meeting may be

called at any time, by any member of the IEP team, to make these revisions. The child must be evaluated at a minimum of every 3 years to determine if the child continues to qualify as a "child with a disability" and their current educational needs.

Components of the IEP

Now that we have discussed the steps involved in creating the IEP, we outline the specific components, along with the purpose for each. One thing that is important to keep in mind regarding IEPs is that even though they must contain the same basic information, the format may look different from state to state. In researching information from various regions across the country, we found that many states provide copies of their IEP forms on the state's department of education website. What we also found is that, with a few exceptions, most of the forms follow roughly the same format. Thus, although the IEP format will vary within and across states, there are standard criteria that must be included, regardless of where the document is being written. According to the U.S. Department of Education website, the IEP contains the following basic components:

- **Student Profile/Present Level of Educational Performance (PLEP):** This section outlines biographical data of the student, how the student is performing academically, and a description of the student's speech and/or language deficits. Information may come from tests, classroom assignments, or teacher/parent observations.
- **Progress Reporting:** This section states the frequency and method as to how parents will be informed of the student's progress (written reports, phone calls, conferences).
- **Special Instructional Factors:** This section is for the purpose of identifying if the student has any limitations that will impede his or her learning, such as hearing or visual impairment, limited English proficiency, the need for assistive technology, or adaptive physical education.
- **Transition Services:** This section is designed to address the needs of students in high school in order to implement programs that will enable them to transition from school to a vocational setting or postsecondary education (the age of transition varies from state to state, and can start as early as 14 years). Transition information must address the following areas: (a) recreation and leisure; (b) community participation; (c) postsecondary training and learning opportunities; (d) home living; and (e) work (job and job training). When a child is age 16, the IEP is required to document any needed transition services for preparing the child to leave the school environment.
- **Transfer of Rights:** This section informs the parent/student that all rights pertaining to special education services transfer to the student at age 18 years. The date the student was notified of the transfer of rights must be indicated in this section of the IEP. A minimum of a year prior to the age of majority, the IEP should state that the student has been notified of any rights that will transfer to him or her. Parents must be given a *Notice of Transfer of Parental Rights*.

▪ **Goals:** These include broad statements that describe what a student can reasonably be expected to accomplish within a 12-month period of time in a special education program. Goals focus on academic skills or social/physical needs, must be related to the child's PLEP, and must be measurable. They must include the student's present level and expected level of performance.

▪ **Benchmarks:** Also known as goals, benchmarks are measurable, intermediate steps leading to the attainment of the goal. There must be at least two benchmarks per goal, and they must include the following: skill/behavior, conditions, criteria, and evaluation methods similar to our earlier discussion of behavioral goals. The IEP includes how often how the child's progress will be assessed and how the parents will be notified of their progress.

▪ **Special Education and Related Services:** In this section you will find the type of service being provided (speech therapy) and the anticipated frequency, duration, location, and beginning and ending date of services. This section also includes, if necessary, supplementary aids and services, accommodations needed for assessments, assistive technology, and any other related services.

▪ **Extended School Year (ESY):** The term *extended school year* encompasses a range of options in providing programs in excess of the traditional 180-day school year, due to issues of regression (loss of skills during an absence of intervention) and recoupment (recovering skills that were lost). In most cases, the IEP team will meet to determine if a student is eligible for ESY and make the appropriate recommendations.

▪ **Least Restrictive Environment (LRE):** Refers to the amount of time a student with a disability will participate in the regular classroom with nondisabled peers. An explanation of when and why the student will be excluded from the regular classroom is required.

▪ **Signature Section:** The signature of everyone in attendance at the IEP meeting, or who will participate in carrying out the student's IEP, is found in this section. There are generally specific titles listed, such as parent, local educational agency (LEA) representative, special education teacher, general education teacher, student, and other agency representative. There is space for other names to be added, if necessary.

Individualized Family Services Plan (IFSP)

The IFSP came about as a result of *The Program for Infants and Toddlers with Disabilities,* or Part C of IDEA. Part C is a federal grant program that assists states in operating a comprehensive statewide program or early intervention services for infants and toddlers with disabilities, serving children from birth through age 3 years and their families. The program was originally established by Congress in 1986 in recognition of "an urgent and substantial need" to enhance the development of infants and toddlers with disabilities; reduce educational costs by minimizing the need for special education through early intervention; minimize the likelihood of institutionalization and maximize independent living; and enhance the capacity of families to meet their child's needs. Children served under Part C of IDEA are those with developmental delay "as measured by appropriate diagnostic instruments and procedures," including (a) cognitive development; (b) physical development, including vision and hearing; (c) communication development; (d) social or emotional development; and (e) adaptive development (IDEA, 2004). An IFSP documents and guides the early intervention process for children with disabilities and their families. It is the vehicle through which effective early intervention is implemented in accordance with Part C of the IDEA. It contains information about the services necessary to facilitate a child's development and enhance the family's capacity to facilitate the child's development. Through this process, family members and service providers work as a team to plan, implement, and evaluate services tailored to the family's unique concerns, priorities, and resources (IDEA, 2004).

How Is the IFSP Different From the IEP?

There are several factors that distinguish the IEP from the IFSP, but the most noticeable difference is the inclusion of the word *family*. The name *Individualized Family Service Plan* was chosen because the family is the constant in a child's life and is therefore the focus of the intervention plan. According to the Council for Exceptional Children, there are several ways in which the IFSP differs from the IEP:

- It includes outcomes targeted for the family, as opposed to focusing only on the eligible child.
- It includes the notion of natural environments, which encompass

home or community settings. This focus creates opportunities for learning interventions in everyday routines and activities, rather than only in formal, contrived environments.
- It includes activities undertaken with multiple agencies beyond the scope of Part C (see explanation above). These are included to integrate all services into one plan.
- It names a service coordinator to help the family during the development, implementation, and evaluation of the IFSP.

The family's concerns, priorities, and resources guide the entire IFSP process. Early intervention should be seen as a system of services and supports available to families to enhance their capacity to care for their children.

There are also several ways that the IFSP is similar to the IEP. As noted in the section on the IEP, you will find that an IFSP also has the following:

- A statement of the child's present levels of development
- A statement of the family's strengths and needs related to enhancing the child's development
- A statement of major outcomes expected to be achieved for the child and family
- The criteria, procedures, and timelines for determining progress
- The specific early intervention services necessary to meet the unique needs of the child and the family, including the frequency, intensity, and method of delivery
- The natural environment(s) in which services will be provided, including justification, if any, of why the

services will not be provided in a natural environment

- The projected dates for initiation of services and their anticipated duration
- Name of the service provider who is responsible for implementing the plan and coordinating with other agencies
- Steps to support the child's transition to preschool or other appropriate services

One thing that you can see from the above goals of the IFSP is the importance of goal setting. Note that it mentions specific goals, ways to measure them, and who will measure progress. Examples of an IEP, IFSP, and the corresponding forms may be found on each state's website (Nebraska, http://www.ifspweb.org/forms.html; Alabama, http://www.alsde.edu/sec/ses/Pages/home.aspx).

How Does the IEP Reflect Specific Goals?

Any child who has an IEP will have specific annual goals and benchmarks to go along with those goals for every area in which he or she is receiving special education services, such as reading, math, language, and speech.

You may be asking yourself, what is an annual goal? What is a benchmark? These and other questions are answered in this section, as we explore the world of goal writing in the public schools.

We have been talking about long-term and short-term goals and up until this point have not mentioned anything about benchmarks. The reason for this is that the term *benchmark* is relative only to IEP paperwork. To provide a brief definition, *benchmarks are major milestones that specify skill or performance levels a student needs to accomplish toward reaching his or her annual goal.* You might be thinking that this is similar to the definition of a short-term goal, and you are correct. Depending on the state, either benchmarks or short-term goals or both are used interchangeably on the IEP. For example, according to the Nebraska Department of Education website, a benchmark represents the actual content or performance the student is to accomplish at a specific interval or grade level. It defines a short-term goal as a measurable, intermediate step between a student's present level of educational performance (PLEP) and the annual goals established for the student (Nebraska, 2014). In the state of New Mexico, the goals page is titled, "Annual Goals and Short-Term Goals or Benchmarks." In Tennessee, the same page is titled, "Measurable Annual Goals and Benchmarks/Short-term Instructional Goals for IEP/Transition Activities," and in California, the page is simply titled, "Annual Goals and Goals." Keep in mind that there are software programs that generate IEPs, and many school systems use these. Based on state requirements, school system policies, and how goals are written, you simply fill in the student's information, and the IEP will be generated for you.

Both benchmarks and short-term goals are developed based on a logical breakdown of the annual goal and guide the development and modification, as necessary, of strategies that will be most effective in realizing the goals. Goals provide a system for measuring the student's progress toward long-range expectations. After the IEP team develops measurable goals for a student, it must develop effective strategies to realize those goals and measurable, intermediate steps (short-term goals) or major milestones (benchmarks) that enable families, students, and educators to monitor progress.

Below you will find some examples of annual goals and benchmarks from two students. We will start with each student's present level of academic achievement and functional performance (PLAAFP) and then include annual goals and benchmarks to support the annual goal.

Student 1

PLAAFP: Nakaiyah has language deficits that impact her in the classroom. Currently, Nakaiyah is able to answer basic comprehension questions about reading passages as well as inferential "why" questions. She is able to identify and define new vocabulary words using context clues as a strategy for enhancing her understanding of the word. Although Nakaiyah does well with vocabulary in reading, Nakaiyah is having difficulties learning and applying academic vocabulary. She also still has difficulties with producing concise, accurate summaries of information she has read. These language deficits are negatively impacting her performance across the general education curriculum.

Measurable Annual Goal: By March 2016, Nakaiyah will demonstrate increased receptive and expressive language skills by determining the main idea and relevant, supporting details in a text to produce a summary of the text [ELA 6.12.3] on four out of five opportunities, and identifying and providing definitions of academic vocabulary words [ELA 6.42.2] with 80% accuracy on given opportunities.

Benchmarks:
1. By May 2015, Nakaiyah will determine the main idea and one relevant, supporting detail in a text to produce a summary of the text [ELA 6.12.3] on four out of five opportunities.
2. By October 2015, Nakaiyah will determine the main idea and three relevant, supporting details in a text to produce a summary of the text [ELA 6.12.3] on four out of five opportunities.
3. By December 2015, Nakaiyah will identify the definition of academic and tier 1 vocabulary words from a choice of four with 80% accuracy on given opportunities [ELA 6.42.2].
4. By March 2016, Nakaiyah will provide a written or verbal definition for academic and tier 1 vocabulary words with 80% accuracy on given opportunities [ELA 6.42.2].

Student 2

PLAAFP: Billy is a hard worker and is motivated to practice his articulation skills outside the therapy room. This has helped him be successful over the past year. Billy completed articulation testing as part of his 3-year re-evaluation. His articulation testing showed errors at the word level on /SH/. Observation and data collection also indicate that Billy struggles to produce vocalic /R/ (AR, ER, OR, IRE, AIR, and EAR). Billy does have some oral-motor deficits including asymmetrical movement of the lips in retraction and difficulty protruding and rounding his lips. These deficits contribute in part to his articulation errors but he is stimulable for some vocalic /R/ productions as well as /SH/. Billy's articulation errors negatively impact his general education participation because they make it difficult for his teachers and peers to understand him at times in the classroom while reading, answering questions, or participating in conversations.

Measurable Annual Goal: By February 2016, Billy will improve his ability to participate in discussions in the general education classroom by producing /SH/ and /CH/ at the conversation level and vocalic /R/ (AR, ER, OR, AIR, EAR, and IRE) in reading tasks with 80% accuracy [ELA 6.34.4].

Benchmarks:
1. By May 2015, Billy will produce /SH/ and /CH/ in all positions of words during reading tasks with 80% accuracy.
2. By October 2015, Billy will produce vocalic /R/ (AR, ER, OR, AIR, EAR, and IRE) in all positions of words during sentence tasks with 80% accuracy.
3. By December 2015, Billy will produce vocalic /R/ (AR, ER, OR, AIR, EAR, and IRE) in all positions of words during reading tasks with 80% accuracy.
4. By February 2016, Billy will produce /SH/ and /CH/ in all positions of words during conversation tasks with 80% accuracy.

Measurable Annual Goal: David will eliminate use of final consonant deletion by producing the target phonemes /p,m,n,b,k,g,d,t/ in the final position with 90% accuracy in structured oral activities in his preschool classroom as measured by SLP progress monitoring.

Benchmarks:
1. By the end of the first 9 weeks, David will imitate the target

phonemes at the word level with 80% accuracy.
2. By the end of the second 9 weeks, David will produce the target phonemes at the spontaneous word level with 80% accuracy.
3. By the end of the third 9 weeks, David will produce the target phonemes at the spontaneous phrase/sentence level with 80% accuracy.
4. By the end of the fourth 9 weeks, David will produce the target phonemes in structured oral activities with 90% accuracy.

As you can see, goals, benchmarks, and goals are written quite differently across states, and it will be up to you to familiarize yourself with your school's process.

Similarities and Differences in Goal-Writing Across Settings

Table 6–2 illustrates goal writing similarities and differences across university, medical, and educational settings. We first remind you about similarities. First, every work setting requires that goals are set and that they are written down in some format. Second, the goals must be measurable and time specific. A third similarity is that in all settings the SLP is required to take periodic measurements to determine if the client is making progress toward the goal that was initially set. Fourth, documentation is viewed as critical in all work settings. Finally, the functional relevance of goals is important in all work settings.

Regardless of the setting, your goals and benchmarks must be written so they can pass the "stranger test." In other words,

Table 6–2. Goal Writing Across Work Settings

Goal Writing Similarities		
Established goals are required		
Goals must be written behaviorally		
Functional relevance of goals is optimal		
Documentation of progress is important		
Periodic measurement is required to determine progress toward goals		
Goal Writing Differences		
University	**Medical**	**School**
Not team oriented	Team oriented	Team oriented
Goals written in client folder	Goals written in patient chart	Goals written in IEP
Goals may be functional	Goals must be functional and related to FIM scores	Goals are educationally based
Extensive data samples	Smaller data samples	Moderate data samples
Goals can be changed quickly	Goals can be changed quickly	Difficult to change goals without IEP meeting
Goals are for the semester	Goals often for short time periods	Goals are annual with periodic benchmarks

they should be written so that someone who did not write them could use them to develop appropriate instructional plans and assess student progress. They should also be written to pass the "so what? test," meaning the patient or client's team understands the rationale and importance of the goal or benchmark. The team would pose the question, "Is the skill indicated in this goal or benchmark really an important skill for the patient to learn?" If the answer is "No," then most likely, the goal is not appropriate.

Goal-setting differences across work settings revolve around several issues. First, there can be more or less involvement of multidisciplinary teams in developing goals. This is more important in medical and school settings than in the university clinic. The place where goals are written down is

a second difference among settings. In the university setting, we write goals in treatment plans or reports that are placed in a client's folder. In medical settings, the goals are part of a patient's medical chart. In school systems, the IEP is the place to write goals. A third difference in goal writing is the length and form of the goal statements. In the university setting, goals are written in narrative form and tend to be lengthier than in other settings. In the medical setting, goals are brief and there is liberal use of medical abbreviations. Goals in school systems are often midway between university and medical settings in length. A fourth difference among settings is the length of the sample gathered to verify progress toward goals. In the university, it is not unusual for students to take language samples several times during a semester to verify progress. On the other hand, medical settings use short tasks and FIM scores to monitor patient progress. School systems, again, are midway between medical settings and university clinics. They often monitor progress with nonstandardized tasks but also give standardized assessments on an annual basis to see if change has occurred. A fifth difference among settings is the presence of a written rationale for goals. In the university setting, students are given practice in developing rationales as part of their goals when they are first beginning practicum. Rationales are almost never seen in the documentation produced by medical facilities and school systems. A sixth difference among settings is the ability to easily change goals. In medical facilities the use of reimbursement codes and oversight by the medical establishment may make it difficult to change goals quickly. In the school setting it may require the IEP team to reconvene to discuss changes in goals. The university clinic can change goals whenever the practicum supervisor feels it is necessary.

It is also important to mention electronic documentation again in this section. Not only do software programs generate diagnostic reports; they can also create progress reports, treatment plans, and discharge notes. Depending on the facility, you may find that you are writing reports on your own or that all you do is enter the client data into a computer and the report is generated for you. Either way, you still have to discern what information is pertinent and where to write it. It is our hope that the information in this book is helpful and that you will gain valuable insight to utilize during your clinical practicum experiences. Our discussion of goal writing has attempted to introduce the practicum student to the elements of well-crafted goals that apply to any work environment. We have also tried to alert students to the changes in goal writing that will be encountered as they do clinical practicum across different types of settings. Goal writing at each facility will be tailored to the client's specific needs, whether they are focused on academic needs or needs they encounter every day (functional). Wherever your clinical training and career lead you, enjoy the challenge of creating meaningful and functional goals to structure therapy to improve the lives of those you serve.

7

Short-Term Progress Reports

Student: "I tried to write down my data in the progress note so that it makes sense. Why is this so important, anyway? I know he's making progress—isn't that all that matters?"

Supervisor: "Of course it matters that he's making progress, but you need to have the right documentation to back it up to the insurance company."

Ah, the real world . . . the place where money is the name of the game—at least, that is, if you are talking about the real world of hospitals, nursing homes, or a private practice. Here, billing policies, copayments, insurance claims, and reimbursement are an everyday part of life. Patients must pay for services, and in most cases, their health insurance, whether it is Medicare, Medicaid, or private, will cover a portion of the cost.

There are places, however, where this is not the case. Take for instance, the public schools. There, you do not have to worry about establishing fees for your services, filing insurance claims, or methods of payment. And unless you work in a school system that bills Medicaid, you do not have to worry about payments for services at all.

Yes, it is true that in many parts of the real world, you will not get paid if you do not have the adequate documentation to support what you are doing in therapy. But it is also true that even in the world of the university clinic, which some will claim is not "the real world," you learn to report on your clients' progress because it is an integral part of the therapy process—not just because you will not get paid. You would think a doctor was crazy if he or she put you on medication for an infection and then commented, "Well, we just thought we'd try those pills for the heck of it. We don't really care what effect they're having." Reporting the progress of your clients and/or patients is paramount to a successful course of treatment. According to Paul (1994), "Clear and comprehensive records are necessary to justify the need for treatment, to document the effectiveness of that treatment, and to have a legal record of events." In addition, as cited in Middleton et al. (2001, p. 39), the ASHA Professional Services Board, (ASHA, 1990), which defines standards for clinical service in speech-language pathology, states, "The quality of services provided is evaluated and documented on a systematic and continuing basis." In other words, the only way for you to know if what you are doing in therapy is working is to take accurate data, analyze that data on a daily or weekly basis, and then make modifications accordingly.

At this point, you may be asking yourself, "But how will I know how to do this?" For starters, one of the main purposes of this book is to expose you to the paperwork and reporting requirements you will be expected to master by the time you finish your graduate work. That way, when you are called upon to complete any type of documentation, whether it's related to assessment or treatment, you will at least have an idea of what is expected. In addition, your clinical supervisor(s) will assist you a great deal when you begin your clinical practicum experience. ASHA understands the importance of good supervision when it relates to students in training—so much so, in fact, that it has outlined 13 supervisory "tasks" (Chapter 13) that inform student clinicians of what to expect from their supervisors. These guidelines ensure that all students enrolled in speech-language pathology (SLP) practicum will be guided and directed in all areas of service delivery by a competent, licensed clinician.

Daily Progress Reports

There would be no way to measure the efficacy of your speech-language therapy if not for daily progress reporting. Data taken during each therapy session is used to determine several things: (a) if the client is making progress, (b) that the treatment techniques are appropriate, (c) when modi-

fications need to be made, and (d) how to plan for future sessions.

The SOAP note, as it is affectionately known in the world of SLP, is a staple of daily reporting on client progress. *SOAP* is an acronym that stands for *subjective*, *objective*, *assessment*, and *plan*. SOAP notes are also commonly used by medical and rehabilitation staff and therefore may appear frequently in other sections of medical charts.

The following is a description of each area of the SOAP note and an example of the information contained therein:

Subjective (S): A description of the client's physical and/or emotional state, including affect, mood, level of motivation, attention, and so on. It is also appropriate to report relevant client or family comments.

> **"S" Example 1:** Mr. Jones was in a pleasant mood during therapy today, although he stated that he was a little tired. His wife stated, "He didn't sleep well last night" and he reported difficulty concentrating during the session.

> **"S" Example 2:** Cowan was eager to begin therapy today. She told the clinician, "I've been practicing my new /s/ sound!" Cowan's mother agreed that they had been practicing with their home program.

> **"S" Example 3:** Kirk was noncompliant during therapy today. He frequently replied "No" when asked to participate in therapy activities and required cueing to remain in his seat.

Objective (O): Includes information regarding the target behaviors, session goals, and data for each goal. If testing was done, the name of the test(s) administered and the results should be written. According to Moon-Meyer (2004), *the facts* belong in the objective part of the SOAP note. In addition to your data, you want to include any information that will support a statement made in the subjective part (Moon-Meyer, 2004).

"O" Example 1: The client will improve immediate memory by using chunking to recall six-digit sequences with no cuing and 75% accuracy.

Data: Mr. Jones achieved 4/10 (40%) accuracy on his first attempt. When he was reinstructed with regard to the technique of chunking and the stimuli was repeated, performance increased to 8/10 (80%) accuracy.

"O" Example 2: The client will produce /s/ final in phrases modeled by the clinician while playing a board game with 80% accuracy.

Data: Cowan achieved 17/20 (85%) accuracy today. Cue 2 increased accuracy to 20/20 (100%.)

"O" Example 3: The client will follow two-step directions while subvocalizing with 80% accuracy.

Data: Kirk achieved 2/10 (20%) accuracy. Repeating the stimulus and other cues did not increase accuracy.

Assessment (A): Includes an explanation of what your data mean and factors that may have affected performance. Also includes a note about the type of stimuli, if necessary, and the effectiveness of cues and reinforcement.

"A" Example 1: Mr. Jones's accuracy was decreased from previous

sessions due to reported fatigue and difficulty concentrating. Repeating the stimulus and a verbal cue to chunk the information increased his accuracy significantly.

"A" Example 2: Cowan met criteria for the third consecutive session while using consistent stimuli to target /s/ initial phrases. When cues were needed, the visual cue (mirror) was most effective.

"A" Example 3: Kirk's performance for following directions decreased from previous sessions due to decreased attention and compliance. Kirk's accuracy did not improve when he was provided with cues. Kirk frequently did not attempt to subvocalize and was only able to follow the first part of the direction.

Plan (P): Includes a statement about what is planned for the next treatment session and a rationale. May include reference to goals, cues, reinforcement, and stimuli.

"P" Example 1: Mr. Jones was given homework to practice on a daily basis with his wife. Chunking will continue to be targeted to increase auditory memory. Cues should remain the same due to effectiveness in increasing accuracy.

"P" Example 2: Increase goal to /s/ initial spontaneous phrases while playing "Fish-n-Say." A probe list will be used to assess generalization for other positions. Cues will be restructured based on goal modification. Reinforcement with stickers will be continued due to Cowan's increased motivation.

"P" Example 3: No modifications to the objective or cues will be made due to data not representing Kirk's true abilities. The current objective will be addressed in the next session also. A behavior modification plan will be discussed with Kirk's mom to implement in future sessions to increase compliance and motivation.

Now that we know what is contained in the SOAP note, let's examine what one will look like across the various settings and how they are used in everyday treatment.

The University Setting

As a practicum student in the university clinic, you will serve clients with a variety of diagnoses across the life span. In many university training programs, students are taught to use the SOAP note as the primary tool for data reporting. In our clinic, students write a SOAP note for each session, whether the client comes one, two, or three times per week. This may not be the case in all clinics. In other situations, you may write just one note for the week or after a certain number of sessions. It should be noted that the SOAP note should be concise and detailed, although approved abbreviations can be used, and information does not have to be communicated using complete sentences as long as it is understandable to the person reading the note. It is common that clinics use an electronic medical record (EMR), but if not, progress or SOAP notes will be filed in a confidential and secure place.

In some settings, speech-language pathologists (SLPs) fill out weekly and monthly progress reports; however, this is not usually the case in the university clinic. In gen-eral, the SOAP notes are used to record all of the data for the semester, and then this information is summarized in the end of semester treatment or progress report. For this reason, information contained in the SOAP note must be timely and accurate. Without accurate data documented, it is very difficult to determine if true progress is being made. Let's examine a few SOAP notes from clients in the university clinic.

Example 1: Aphasia Client

Subjective: Mr. Taylor was in a pleasant mood and put forth good effort throughout the session. Mrs. Taylor reported that he is successfully using gestures to communicate his needs when he experiences anomia when speaking with her.

Objective:

STG 1: The client will match a picture to a corresponding written phrase from a field of 3 with no cuing and 70% accuracy.

Data: 11/15 (73%); increased to 13/15 (87%) with field of 2

STG 2: The client will name common household objects with 60% accuracy and semantic cues.

Data: 4/12 (33%;) cues did not increase accuracy

STG 3: The client will provide the missing word in a common phrase with minimal cues from the clinician with 80% accuracy.

Data: 3/10 (30%) with minimal cueing; increased to 7/10 (70%) with the phonemic cue

STG 4: The client will copy the clinician's written model of personal information with 100% accuracy with verbal cues.

Data: 5/5 (100%) with verbal cues

Assessment: Mr. Taylor's reading comprehension improved from last session; however, he continues to exhibit significant anomia during verbal structured and unstructured tasks. He had increased difficulty with confrontational naming today and quickly abandoned the attempt. He required increased time to respond to the phrase completion task, and needed frequent phonemic cues. Criteria have been met for copying personal information over the past three sessions; this goal will be modified to increase complexity of this task.

Plan: The current expressive language goals will continue to be targeted and the gestures will be encouraged when he is unable to use a circumlocution. The confrontational naming goal will be modified to decrease the level of difficulty. The stimuli for reading comprehension will be varied to assess generalization. The phonemic cue will be provided first to increase success with common phrases. The written language goal will be modified to target personal information with only a partial model, and corresponding homework will be provided.

Example 2: Child Language Client

Subjective: Max had difficulty remaining in his seat today and required frequent redirection to attend. His mother stated, "He has a lot of energy this morning!"

Objective:

STG 1: The client will respond appropriately to "what" and "where" questions after listening to a four- to five-sentence story with 80% accuracy and no cues.

Data: 10/20 (50%); increased to 15/20 (75%) with repetition of stimuli

STG 2: The client will identify the phoneme when provided with the sound for all short vowels with 100% accuracy and no cues.

Data: 7/10 (70%); increased to 10/10 (100%) when given choice cue

STO 3: The client will read 10 out of 15 sight words when presented on flash cards by the clinician.

Data: 8/15

Assessment: Max's performance on "wh" questions decreased from previous sessions; however, this may be attributed to his high energy level and difficulty focusing. He enjoyed the Bingo game used during the vowel activity, and his accuracy increased to 100% when given a choice cue, indicating improvement from the previous session. When in error, Max continues to identify /E/ for /I/. He exhibited hesitation recognizing sight words, although today was the first session these words were targeted. He became easily distracted throughout the session, so he may benefit from more frequent breaks.

Plan: "What" and "where" questions will continue to be targeted, and repetition will be provided when needed. A cue such as "make sure your listening ears are on" should be implemented prior to reading the story. Short vowels will continue to be targeted, and long vowels will be introduced. The same sight words should be targeted to increase speed of identification and accuracy. Homework will be given for daily practice identifying short vowel names and sounds. A schedule board and high-interest reward to increase attention will be initiated.

Example 3: Child Articulation Client

Subjective: Hannah was eager to begin therapy and was compliant throughout the session. Hannah's mother reported that her teacher said she is understanding more of Hannah's speech.

Objective:

STG 1: The client will produce /k/ in the initial position of words while naming picture cards with 80% accuracy and maximum cues.

Data: 2/12 (17%) with maximum cues

STG 2: The client will produce /f/ in the initial position of words while playing Articulation Bingo with 80% accuracy and verbal cues.

Data: 4/12 (33%); increased to 8/12 (67%) with verbal cue and 10/12 (83%) with full model

Assessment: Hannah had significant difficulty producing /k/ initial in spontaneous words and continues to substitute /t/. She also substituted /t/ for /f/ initial; however, the verbal cue of "put your teeth on your lip" was beneficial. She responded well to stickers and was motivated by a schedule board.

Plan: The goal for /k/ initial will be modified to the syllable level to determine a facilitating context, and the cueing hierarchy will be modified accordingly. Bingo will continue to be used to target /f/, since Hannah enjoys the game and the phonetic placement presented as first cue. Hannah's mom will be provided with education regarding phonetic placement so she can implement cueing at home. Hannah is motivated by verbal praise and a sticker at the end of each activity, so that will be continued as reinforcement.

Example 4: Fluency Client

Subjective: Doug was in a good mood today and was excited about the upcoming spring break. He reported that he ordered from a drive-through this weekend and was able to control his rate and maintain his fluency.

Objective:

STG 1: The client will utilize smooth controlled speech during a structured reading task (words, phrases, sentences) with 80% accuracy and minimal cuing.

Data: 9/10 = 90% (words)
6/10 = 60% (phrases)
6/10 = 60% (sentences)

STG 2: The client will reduce disfluencies to less than 20% during a 3-minute conversation with a familiar person in the therapy room.

Data: (15/80) 19%

STO 3: The client will reduce disfluencies to less than 20% when speaking to an unfamiliar person in the therapy room.

Data: (100/386) 26% in 10 minutes of conversation

Assessment: Doug's reading at the phrase and sentence level was not as fluent as in previous sessions. He stated that he did not focus on being "as relaxed as he should have." He still felt that overall, "it was pretty good." He had difficulty when speaking with Alex, an unfamiliar person, and admitted that his blocks were longer and more frequent because he was not using his techniques. He appears to be motivated by tracking his progress on a weekly graph.

Plan: The next session will be recorded to allow for feedback and as a basis for discussion about his self-monitoring skills. Stimuli will be selected for reading that do not contain problematic words in order to increase success. Doug will continue to be provided opportunities to speak with unfamiliar persons to practice his techniques.

These are just a few examples of what a SOAP note looks like. As mentioned previously, the SOAP format is used in many different settings and will vary in length, detail, and content, depending on the setting. Additional examples of SOAP notes are included in Appendix I.

The Medical Setting

Many of the medical professionals we interviewed informed us that students are often timid or hesitant when writing information in a patient's chart. They seem to be afraid of writing the wrong information, writing too much information, or not writing enough information. It is our goal to help you know what to write and how to write it.

As mentioned previously, SOAP notes are standard documentation for many different medical professionals. In a hospital, skilled nursing facility, or rehabilitation center, doctors, nurses, and rehab staff (therapists) may all use SOAP notes to communicate regarding a patient's care. Therefore, many of the SOAP notes found in a patient's chart may look similar. Within the SOAP note, terminology and goals will vary among professions and across settings. We feel it is worth explaining a few terms, abbreviations, and symbols that you may encounter in a medical setting. Appendix F lists commonly used symbols and abbreviations and their meanings. Due to the limited amount of space, as well as the number of professionals who add information to a patient's medical chart, you can appreciate the need for the SLP in a medical setting to use abbreviations and symbols as often as possible.

Because patients requiring SLP services at a medical facility have likely recently experienced one or more major medical events, have multiple diagnoses, or have multiple comorbidities, you will be using abbreviations outside of those related to communication skills. When working in a medical facility, you are strongly warned to only use approved abbreviations so all those reading the chart will understand precisely what you are communicating. For example, if you are recommending that a patient be "NPO" due to severe dysphagia, you want to be sure to use the appropriate abbreviation so as not to misconstrue this information and endanger your patient. In addition to using abbreviations in your paperwork, you need to identify abbreviations when reading about your patient in the chart. Understanding abbreviations is vital when making evaluation and treatment decisions about your patient. Learning abbreviations for medical conditions such as COPD (chronic obstructive pulmonary disease) and GERD (gastroesophageal reflux disease) is important as this might indicate a need for a swallowing evaluation. When you encounter an abbreviation with which you are not familiar, do not risk guessing but take the time to look up the term or ask your supervisor. There is typically a dictionary of medical abbreviations and terms at the nurses' station.

Depending on the facility, terminology used in documentation may vary based on the type of system used to measure a patient's progress. As we mentioned in Chapter 6, it is common to see *functional independence measures* or FIM scores. This system, as the name implies, evaluates patients based on their level of independence in a variety of areas.

We have found that most facilities use this system or one that is similar. Some facilities may only use the numbers from the FIM scale or similar abbreviations. For instance, they may write, "Pt. will improve comprehension from level 4 to level 5," or they may use MOD or MIN rather than MIN-A (minimum assistance) or MOD-I (modified independent). In general, the criteria are the same even if the abbreviations vary. Let's take a look at what a SLP note might actually look like in a rehabilitation setting. The following SOAP note is for a patient who is working on memory, intelligibility, and problem solving using a FIM rating.

> **Subjective:** Pt seen for 2 units of speech tx today; pt alert & cooperative with no complaint of pain.
>
> **Objective:** Pt completed 15 trials of OMEs with SPV, to ↑ labial and lingual ROM. Pt able to recall 2/3 speech strategies and completed speech intelligibility tasks at the imitative sentence level with MIN-A. Pt required mod cues to provide solutions for 8/10 problems related to ADLs.
>
> **Assessment:** Independence with OMEs ↑ today, less cueing was needed for intelligibility tasks, and increased cueing needed for problem-solving tasks, as situations were more complex.
>
> **Plan:** Continue POC.

Due to daily caseload numbers, lack of space in the medical chart, and the number of people who have to read the information, most speech pathology notes in a medical setting are brief and use similar terminology. This is true for other therapists as well as nurses, doctors, and other professional staff, making it even more important that the SLP in a medical setting become familiar with all types of terminology. It is vital that you only use approved abbreviations, as using an abbreviation that someone else is unfamiliar with may result in confusion and a failure to communicate.

Keep in mind that as a student clinician, when you sign any documentation, a licensed SLP will be required to sign as well. Therefore, even if you are unsure about what to write, your supervisor will review and sign off on your note. When learning how to best document your patient's goals and progress, you should remember the common adage, "If it is not written in the patient's chart, it didn't happen." While your notes and reports will not be as lengthy as in the university clinic, it is still vital to document certain aspects of evaluation and treatment. Wherever you are placed, you should take the time to become familiar with the facility's method of writing goals. Different facilities have different requirements, and there are typically very specific guidelines based on third-party payer requirements.

The School Setting

Due to the federally mandated use of the Individualized Education Program (IEP), the SOAP note is not a staple of reporting in the public schools. Most SLPs who work in the public schools devise their own system to track data and simply report final data in the section of the IEP form that is designated specifically for reporting progress. Methods of data collection may vary greatly among school systems, schools within the same system, or individual therapists. As a practicum student in the public schools, you will be expected to follow the system that your particular school has in place. This may mean that you will use specific data collection forms or that you design your own form; each school will be different.

Even though forms and procedures may differ across school systems, what remains the same is how each child's progress is reported on the actual IEP form. This is federally mandated, and therefore not open to interpretation. Progress reporting is a necessary component of the delivery of SLP services. Becoming efficient at reporting progress or lack thereof, regardless of the setting in which you eventually practice, is a crucial skill to develop as a student clinician and one that will only enhance your clinical skills throughout your professional career.

8

Long-Term Progress Reports

Our goal as speech-language pathologists is to help our clients attain (to the greatest extent possible) normal function of their speech, language, or swallowing abilities. In order to accomplish this task, we must gather reliable data that measure and validate this change over time. As we have discussed in previous chapters, these data are what determines if we have achieved our goals through the delivery of speech-language pathology services, as well as our ability to receive payment or reimbursement (from a third-party payer) for those services. Now that we have shown you how to write goals, objectives, daily notes, and short-term progress reports, we would be remiss if we did not discuss how to report progress for patients who are in therapy for an extended period of time. Long-term progress reports summarize information that has most likely been documented in previous documentation such as daily notes and/or short-term progress notes. This chapter provides setting-specific information on long-term progress reports as well as information about discharge summaries, when they are needed, and what they look like.

The University Setting

Due to the nature of how treatment takes place in a university clinic, namely, that clients receive treatment for the duration of a quarter or semester, a long-term progress report generally serves as a summary for the therapy term. In addition to the daily SOAP or weekly progress notes, most training programs require students to prepare a final report that includes data for all of the client's goals for the entire term. This document may be referred to as a *Final Treatment Report* or *Semester Progress Report*, depending on the university program and the terminology it chooses to use. Most clients who attend a university clinic for speech-language services expect these reports, as do other allied professionals who collaborate with clinicians in university clinics.

For example, if a child is receiving services in the public school as well as at the university clinic, a copy of the semester progress report is usually sent to the school SLP in order to ensure that both parties are addressing the same needs for the child. Also, if a client has been referred to the university clinic by another professional (psychologist, physician, occupational therapist, etc.), it is standard practice to send that individual a copy of the client's progress report with a note thanking him or her for the referral. If a client is being seen by a number of different professionals, this sharing of information can be vital in the overall treatment of the client.

The long-term progress report is important for several reasons:

1. *Short-term and long-term progress reporting are required by ASHA and third-party payers.* All university programs must abide by certain ASHA guidelines in order to maintain their accreditation. These guidelines stipulate that a variety of documentation must be in place on a consistent basis. Students must keep an accurate record of their clinical hours, and there must be a system in place to keep up with each client's progress. Most clinics have a confidential file system, in which each client has a personal and confidential file that is kept in a secure location, or in an electronic medical record (EMR). At the end of each term, progress reports must be placed or scanned into the client's file for safekeeping. ASHA requires this confidential filing system, as does the federal government, due to enactment of the Health Information Portability and Accountability Act (HIPAA). As far as billing is concerned, if a clinic bills Medicaid, Medicare, or private insurance, accurate records ensure that these entities are being billed for valid service delivery. Any discrepancies in paperwork can result in denial of payment for services, and this reflects poorly on the program, the clinic, and the university.

2. *Clients may remain in therapy for several semesters, or even years, and a record should be kept of past performance.* It is not uncommon for many patients (especially adults) in a university clinic to end up there due to an insurance company being unwilling to continue paying for services through a hospital or private practitioner. As we discussed in an earlier chapter, third-party payers usually stipulate the exact number of sessions they will cover relating to any type of rehabilitation therapy. Once the patient has completed the designated number of sessions, he or she must find services elsewhere or pay out-of-pocket expenses. And, due to the fact that university clinics are training facilities, many operate on a sliding fee scale, based on a client's income. It is also necessary that students have clients for whom they can provide services in order for the clinical training program to thrive. Therefore, some clients will remain in therapy for an extended period of time due to the reduced or waived fees and willingness of the clinical staff at the university clinic to work with them.

3. *Clients often have a new student clinician each semester, and historical data are important when planning treatment each term.* Most university training programs have the goal of providing student clinicians with the most diverse clinical experience possible, allowing them to work with both children and adults in a variety of disorder areas. This is usually accomplished through practicum experience in the university clinic as well as off-campus sites. It is for this reason that clients are often seen in the university clinic who have been discharged from other private practitioners, hospitals, or rehabilita-

tion facilities, due to insurance reasons or lack of progress. Generally, clients in the university clinic will have a new student clinician each semester in order for students to receive training in all disorder areas. This is especially true for a client with a less common disorder. In order for the new clinician to best prepare to treat the client, a thorough review of previous long-term reports is necessary. This sheds light on what progress has been made or lack thereof, and the use of certain therapy approaches, cues, reinforcement, and procedures. Much time can be saved when attempting to craft the most efficient and effective treatment plan by reviewing long-term reports.

4. *The client and/or parent or caregiver is provided with a record of progress.* Just as you expect a report from a physician or specialist when you have any type of testing or treatment done, your clients expect the same information regarding the speech therapy services you have provided. Not only are clients/parents given progress reports in order to summarize data for themselves or their child's therapy sessions, in the case of older children and adults, but the progress report may serve as a tool to motivate the clients to continue with therapy until maximum potential is achieved.

It is important to add here that many times, the long-term progress report will also serve as a discharge summary. If a client is being discharged from therapy, this is usually mentioned in the "Recommendations" section of the report. For example, "Based on Mr. Smith meeting criteria over the past three sessions, it is recommended that he be discharged from speech therapy at this time." More than likely, your clinic will have protocols in place for how and when to write progress/treatment reports, and your clinical supervisors will assist you in this process. However, we provide an example of a university clinic long-term treatment report in Appendix G.

The Medical Setting

Due to the nature of treatment across various medical settings, we address each one separately in this section.

The Rehabilitation Setting

As we mentioned in Chapter 4, patients are typically admitted to a rehabilitation hospital for a predetermined amount of time. This depends on the patient's level of functioning, often referred to as *burden of care*, as well as their insurance coverage. Persons aged 65 or older are eligible for Medicare, whereas patients under the age of 65 must rely on private insurance or pay expenses out of pocket. The average stay for Medicare patients is 14 days, although patients who have private insurance may stay longer, depending on how much time their insurance company will allow. At the culmination of their stay in the rehabilitation facility, one of three things will happen. They are (a) discharged home or to a caregiver's home, (b) transferred to the hospital, or (c) admitted to a long-term care facility.

As was evident in the chapter on writing long-term and short-term goals, some facilities do not even bother to write long-term goals, although others have a long-term goal, but the outcomes reflect what one could reasonably expect to accomplish during a 2-week period. For example, a client in a university clinic may have a long-term goal of returning to work on a part-time basis following a stroke or TBI, whereas this same individual may have a long-term goal of following multistep directions with minimal assistance while in the rehabilitation facility. You may want to refer back to Chapter 6 for examples of long-term goals for each type of medical facility. The progress report for these patients will reflect not only the goals that were targeted, but also the amount of time the patient spends working on these goals.

A long-term progress report may also serve as the discharge report for a patient who has only spent 14 days in a rehabilitation facility. The discharge summary may be the same form that was used for reporting the patient's progress and will also use functional independence measures (FIM) scores to indicate the patient's status at discharge. At times, the SLP may actually discharge a patient from speech and language therapy before he or she is discharged from a facility. Whenever the client is discharged from SLP services, whether during his or her stay or at the conclusion, you will generally write a *discharge note or summary* on a specific form. Along with discharge instructions, you may fill out a Patient Education section that indicates what information you have provided to the patient regarding any necessary home care or home program.

The Hospital Setting

Similar to the rehabilitation setting, a patient's stay in a hospital may be very limited. Very often, patients are seen in acute care for just a few days until they are stable enough to be moved to the rehabilitation wing of the hospital, another rehabilitation facility, or discharged home. As a general rule, patients do not have long-term goals in acute care; it is the goal of the medical professionals working with patients in acute care to

get them medically stable so that they can participate in and benefit from any therapies they may need once they recover. The SLP who sees a critically ill patient in acute care may be there only to do a bedside swallowing evaluation to determine if the patient is safe to eat a normal diet, needs diet modifications, or needs alternative means of nutrition.

Once the patient is stable, the physician will write an order for the SLP evaluation. Once this evaluation has been completed and the patient's needs are determined, the SLP will then write appropriate goals for the patient and begin treatment. You may refer back to Chapter 6 for examples of short-term and long-term goals in a hospital setting.

Long-Term Care/ Skilled Nursing Facility

Unless they have been temporarily transferred to the nursing home until they recover enough function to return home, most patients who are in long-term care may remain there for the duration of their life. Even though these patients may remain in the long-term care facility a very long time, they will only qualify for speech-language therapy for a specific amount of time. Therefore, long-term progress reports for these patients are similar to those of the acute care or rehabilitation hospital. The SLP often uses appropriate goals from a *goal bank* and then selects short-term objectives as a way to achieve the long-term goal. Once again, goals must be functional in order for the facility to be reimbursed by Medicare or other third-party payers—if the patient is not making progress, the case cannot be made that he or she should continue receiving services. The long-term goal will most likely be written so that it may be achieved in the time frame that has been stipulated by payment for services.

The School Setting

If you find yourself assigned to a practicum in the public schools, you will become familiar with the *Individualized Education Program* (IEP). With the information provided in Chapter 5, along with the experience you gain firsthand, you will begin to develop an understanding of how the IEP functions. The IEP has a built-in system for tracking progress. Recall from Chapter 6 that for each long-term goal, benchmarks are developed that stipulate a time frame for each goal to be achieved. Personnel responsible for implementing the IEP must then report the student's progress to the parent or guardian of the child who is receiving services on a regular basis. Due to the nature of this periodic reporting system, there is no long-term progress report for children who are being served through the public schools—progress is reported at various intervals throughout the school year, such as every 6 or 9 weeks, and then the parent(s), teachers, special education teachers, and other professionals meet once a year to discuss how the child has progressed based on the benchmarks set forth from the previous year's meeting. In this way, each person who is responsible for implementing the IEP will understand the ultimate academic goal for this child.

It is probably fairly clear to you now that reporting progress is a mainstay in the field of SLP. Without reports of how our clients are performing, we have no way to determine if we should stay the course, modify treatment, or discharge someone from therapy altogether. The long-term progress report tells us if the long-term goal (the ultimate outcome we want for our clients) is being achieved, and if not, how we should proceed in the future.

9

Professional Correspondence

Although we have already discussed many forms of written communication that you will be expected to master during your clinical training, one form that we have not addressed is professional correspondence. In the course of a typical week, the speech-language pathologist (SLP) will generate different types of correspondence in addition to the report writing we have discussed in previous chapters. Whether you are writing referral letters, cover letters, thank-you letters, or e-mails, the ability to communicate effectively will speak volumes about your knowledge, clinical competence, organization, and professionalism. In short, you have the opportunity to establish credibility by using professional and well-written communication. A focus on professionalism should not just be considered in verbal interactions and clinical reports. It should be communicated in our written correspondence as well.

How does your written communication project an image of you? Imagine, if you will, that you are a parent whose child is receiving speech-language therapy at the university clinic. You receive a letter from the student who has been working with your child, and in the first paragraph, there are two typographical errors and a run-on

sentence. What is your impression going to be? Would you think that this student is professional? Would you wonder if this lack of attention to detail might carry over to the student's preparation and competence in providing therapy services for your child? The way we communicate, whether verbally or in writing, truly says a lot about us as professionals.

During your time in school, you will be required to demonstrate two types of writing: academic and clinical. Academic writing may include research papers, journal reviews, case presentations, or answers to comprehensive test questions. Clinical writing encompasses all of the reports and documents we have covered thus far in this text, in addition to the type of correspondence we address in this chapter—e-mails, referral letters, and the like. Although you are expected to come into the university with some basic writing skills that enable you to complete these academic writing tasks, we understand that clinical writing is a unique genre of communication. Students do not come into a training program with knowledge of professional clinical writing. This is a skill you will acquire along with the clinical competencies you develop when becoming a certified SLP.

The Basics

Professional writing is a challenging, yet important and necessary part of your training. Lack of student preparedness in training programs is nothing new, however; the authors have learned through interviews with practicum supervisors and in professional seminars that students' basic writing skills are frequently an area of weakness.

University training programs will address this issue in various ways, and it is our hope that you will have the support you need to become proficient in your professional writing abilities. Unfortunately, there typically is no formal course in clinical writing at most universities, and many students have not received adequate writing practice in general. Although students may have the opportunity to write essays or journal reviews, they do not get any practice with clinical writing until they are thrust into it once they begin the practicum experience. Even then, they are at the mercy of varied supervisors who have different ideas about the level of writing skill they should possess. This is made even more complicated because supervisors may differ in their own styles of clinical writing.

Your university will most likely provide you with sample reports or templates in order to refine your writing skills. Even though writing prowess improves with practice and experience, there is obviously a need for guidelines and examples of what a professionally written document should look like. Middleton et al. (2001) note that making sample reports and training exercises available facilitates the recognition of good writing.

Direct instruction may be provided in courses exclusive to writing or those addressing specific disorders. This can include providing the students with well-written, as well as poorly written sample reports or collaborating with your instructor or classmates to compose a report based on a hypothetical case. Peer response is another avenue to enhance writing skills and critical thinking. It is now widely recognized as a best practice for improved writing. It is not just to improve the final product; it is to improve the students' ability to meta-process. This may be done among peers in your field or within an interdisciplinary curriculum such as nursing, psychology, or social work. The method of peer response usually involves pairs of students exchanging de-identified reports for review. Specific instruction on how to provide feedback in a constructive and professional manner, rather than line editing or "nit-picking" someone else's work forms the basis of the peer response. Students are given a rubric with guiding questions to assist in providing their partner feedback that will result in higher quality documentation, in terms of content, grammar, professional terminology, and attention to detail. Clear guidelines and communication are critical for a beneficial peer response experience.

Format/Organization

All well-written documents must be organized in such a way that makes them easy to follow. How many times have you read and reread something, only to find that you still cannot discern the meaning the writer is attempting to convey? When it comes to drafting a professional document, organization includes everything from sentence structure to word usage to placement of information within the document. Most resources you find that address organizational aspects of professional writing will include a list of "must-haves" for a professional document (Strunk & White, 2000). Many guidelines used in writing business reports include some key components that relate to the business letters, thank-you letters, cover letters, and referral letters discussed in this chapter. In the next section, we provide examples of some of these documents; however, we would like to introduce the following information to you at this time, as we feel it is relevant to organization and it applies to various types of correspondence:

- The letter should be written on letterhead stationery if it is from a clinical facility.
- Every piece of professional correspondence should be dated at the top.
- There should be an address on the letter that includes basic information such as the name, address, and affiliation of the intended recipient of the letter.
- The letter should include a professional and respectful greeting or salutation (e.g., Dear Mrs. Hardy or Dear Dr. Patel).
- The first paragraph of the letter typically provides some background information about the sender so that the recipient of the letter knows something about the person generating the correspondence.
- The body of the letter or memo should contain the reason the document is being written and whom it is written about. It should be broken up into logical paragraphs or subheadings, if necessary.
- There should be a summary or conclusion paragraph reiterating the purpose of the letter and thanking

the recipient for her consideration in reading the document.

- Prior to the signature line there should be what is known as a *complimentary closing* (e.g., "Sincerely, Respectfully").
- The signature line should include the typed name of the sender, her degrees, and position. In the case of students you can refer to yourself as "student clinician," "graduate clinician," and so on.

We will now take a look at how this organizational structure applies to the various types of communication we have mentioned. In general, there are four types of letters that you may be required to write during your clinical training: referral letters, thank-you letters, transmittal (cover) letters, and business letters. These are explained further below:

- **Referral letter:** This will usually accompany a diagnostic or treatment report for a client you are referring to another professional for services not within the scope of practice of the SLP. For example, we routinely refer clients to physicians, psychologists, occupational therapists, physical therapists, special educators, social workers, regular educators, audiologists, among others. This letter describes the reason for the referral and introduces the client to the professional to whom we are referring the case. Without some explanation, the professional would be at a loss to understand the purpose of the referral.
- **Thank-you letter:** This will usually be sent as a follow-up when a

client has been referred to you from another professional. Expressing your appreciation for the referral will hopefully serve to maintain a positive professional relationship and may result in more referrals in the future. Such letters are also used when other professionals donate their time and expertise to consult with you on a case. It is a good policy to thank people for any contributions of time, materials, or finances.

■ **Cover letter:** This usually accompanies a diagnostic or treatment report that is being sent to a professional, client, parent, or caregiver. It is not professional to simply mail a report to someone without a letter of explanation accompanying the document. Such cover letters explain why the report is being sent.

■ **Business letter:** This is used when writing to a company or organization in order to request a service or materials. We also use business letters to correspond with insurance companies and businesses that provide administrative support to clinics such as office supplies, copying machines, and clerical personnel. Business letters might also be used to make other professionals aware of existing clinical programs offered by your facility or announce the establishment of new services by the clinic.

All four of the letters mentioned above require organization, a specific format, and professional communication. The letters sent by the SLP represent not only the individual practitioner, but the facility for which she or he works, so they must be done professionally.

An example of each type of letter is provided below.

Sample Referral Letter

August 2, 2016

Jennifer Palmer, OT
Main Street Rehabilitation
Montgomery, AL

Dear Ms. Palmer:

I am writing this letter in regard to Daniel Lewis, a 3-year-old male, who was seen at this clinic for a speech and language evaluation on July 23, 2016. Daniel was referred to us by his pediatrician due to a speech and language delay. During the case history interview, Janice Lewis, Daniel's mother, also described several other behaviors that are causing her quite a bit of concern.

Based on results of my assessment, Daniel does exhibit a language delay; however, he is also demonstrating self-stimulating behaviors such as repeatedly spinning in circles, as well as diverted eye gaze. Mrs. Lewis reports that Daniel is also a very "picky" eater, and that he "does not like things touching him." Based on results of my evaluation, as well as his mother's concerns, I feel that a comprehensive occupational therapy evaluation is warranted.

I appreciate your assessment of Daniel and am enclosing a copy of our diagnostic report for your review. I look forward to receiving your input on this case.

Sincerely,

Embry Burrus, MCD, CCC/SLP
Speech-Language Pathologist
Auburn University Speech and Hearing Clinic

Enclosure

Sample Thank-You Letter

August 2, 2016

Daniel Rice, M.D.
Regional Medical Clinic
123 Main St.
Auburn, AL 36830

Dear Dr. Rice:

Thank you for referring James Goodwin to our clinic for a speech and language evaluation. We completed our evaluation of James on July 25, 2015, and have recommended that he receive speech therapy at our clinic for the upcoming semester.

Based on the results of testing and informal assessment, James continues to exhibit language and pragmatic difficulties as a result of the traumatic brain injury he sustained approximately one year ago. Your assessment of his social language skills was extremely informative, and we appreciate your insight into this matter. Since we have received James's authorization, we will be happy to send you a progress report at the end of the semester. Should you have any questions, or need further information, please contact us at your convenience.

Once again, thank you for your referral.

Sincerely,

Heather Daniels, BS
Student Clinician
Auburn University Speech &
  Hearing Clinic

Rhonda Wilson, MCD, CCC/SLP
Speech-Language Pathologist
Auburn University Speech &
  Hearing Clinic

Sample Cover Letters

August 7, 2016

Allison Plumb, OT
Main Street Rehabilitation
Montgomery, AL

Dear Ms. Henderson:

Enclosed please find the diagnostic report for Larry Henderson, a 3-year-old male, who was evaluated at this clinic on July 30, 2016. Per our phone conversation, Larry has been referred to your clinic for occupational therapy due to sensory integration disorder and decreased fine motor skills.

Should you need any further information, please contact us at (123) 456-7890. We look forward to hearing from you and collaborating with you in the treatment of this child.

Sincerely,

Amy Sellers, BS   Tim Gosher, MCD, CCC-SLP
Student Clinician   Speech-Language Pathologist
Trinity Speech and Hearing Clinic   Trinity Speech and Hearing Clinic

Enclosure

May 5, 2016

Megan and Michael Carpenter
1199 Ivy Lane
Atlanta, GA 30030

Dear Mr. and Mrs. Carpenter,

Enclosed please find a copy of the treatment report for Daphne from this past semester. I have enjoyed working with Daphne and am proud of how much she has progressed over the past several weeks. Please let me know if you have any questions regarding this report or the home program.

Sincerely,

Marie Peppers   Kelsey Parsons
Graduate Student Clinician   Speech-Language Pathologist
Cauthen Speech and Hearing Clinic   Cauthen Speech and Hearing Clinic

Enclosure

Sample Business Letter

August 7, 2016

Daniel Means, President
Therapy Works, Inc.
123 Main St.
Birmingham, AL

Dear Mr. Means:

My name is Ann Smith, and I am a graduate student in speech-language pathology at Ourtown University. I am very interested in learning more about the therapy materials that you offer for children who have feeding and swallowing disorders. I am about to begin my externship at a pediatric clinic and expect to see a number of children who have been diagnosed with these disorders.

I read in your catalog that a representative from your company will come to our university to demonstrate your products and that you offer a discount if we make a purchase following the demonstration. I would appreciate any assistance you could provide in arranging this for our students.

Thank you for your time and attention to this matter. I may be reached at (123) 456-9900, or via e-mail at a.smith@haleyuniversity.edu. I look forward to hearing from you very soon.

Sincerely,

Ann Smith, BS   Meagan Merrils
Student in SLP   Speech-Language Pathologist
Haley University Speech   Haley University Speech
  and Hearing   and Hearing

Electronic mail is used more often by people communicating in work settings than any other type of written correspondence. Using e-mail may be preferred by many professionals due to the convenience it offers. E-mails will generally serve one of three purposes: (a) transmitting information, (b) requesting information, or (c) requesting or enabling action. We provide a couple of examples in the boxes.

Transmitting Information

Dear Dr. Good,

I am writing in regard to the oral comprehensive exam that I missed due to a death in my family. At your convenience, I would like to meet with you in order to discuss a time to reschedule this exam. Thank you for your understanding and assistance in this matter.

Sincerely,
Rashida King

Dear Mr. Stanley,

I have attached the evaluation report for Charlie Bryce. We were able to administer several standardized tests, as well as make observations during play. Our results, impressions, and recommendations are documented in the report. Please let me know if you have any questions. I hope our assessment can benefit you in your treatment of Charlie.

Sincerely,
Laura Lucas

Requesting Information

Dear Dr. Pardy,

I am contacting you regarding Richie Walters' recent psychological evaluation. I am his current graduate clinician at Premier Speech and Hearing Clinic, and I would greatly appreciate your recommendations on how to manage Richie's behavior in our therapy sessions, based on your recent evaluation of him. I have attached the authorization form from Richie's mother that allows us to share information. At your convenience, please e-mail me a copy of your assessment report. Thank you for your time.

Sincerely,
Regina Morris

Good afternoon Dr. Allen,

My name is Jordan Clover, and I am a student in your Speech Science class. I would like to get a copy of the extra practice worksheet you offered in class. Could you e-mail me the worksheet or let me know when it is convenient to come by your office? I know you said that these concepts build on each other, and I appreciate the opportunity for extra practice.

Thanks,
Jordan Clover

Requesting or Enabling Action

Dear Ms. Jones,

I am writing to inform you that I am in receipt of paperwork from the graduate school that needs to be added to my personal and confidential file. I understand that you only receive information from students at specific times. Please let me know when would be a good time for me to get this information to you. Thank you for your assistance in this matter.

Sincerely,
Beverly Stokes

Good afternoon Mrs. Chilson,

My name is Jody Merchant, and I am Steve Reese's graduate clinician at the Auburn University Speech and Hearing Clinic. I have been able to obtain an authorization form from his father in order to contact you about Steve's communication skills in the classroom. Would you be able to meet with me in order to discuss this? If so, what days and times are best for you? Thank you for your time.

Sincerely,
Jody Merchant

Students have the responsibility of checking their e-mail daily for communications from faculty members or the university administration. It is no excuse to say that you did not read your e-mail if an assignment is given to the class via this form of communication. Often, e-mail is exchanged between facilities for the purpose of scheduling appointments or other tasks associated with clients. In making this point, we would like to add that your e-mails should be just as well written and organized. We emphasize that you should resist the temptation to use "text message" speech, abbreviations, and slang. This will communicate to whomever receives your message a lack of professionalism. Do not make the mistake of communicating something about yourself that you do not intend. It is also wise to remember that any information transmitted electronically is susceptible to eavesdropping by hackers and others, especially if you are communicating over an unsecure connection and using non-encrypted e-mail. As we mentioned in an earlier chapter, you could be violating a client's confidentiality by sending sensitive clinical information by e-mail if it is intercepted by an unintended recipient. Before sending any information electronically, authorization must be obtained. People can also easily access another person's computer and read that person's e-mail or simply look over a shoulder and read the screen. The bottom line is that you must be very careful transmitting client information via e-mail. This also applies to sending clinical reports as e-mail attachments.

SECTION III

Professional Verbal Communication

10

Interacting With Clients and Families

In the previous section of this text we discussed professional written communication in the form of diagnostic reports, treatment plans, and various forms of progress reports. Your written communications have a profound effect on how you are perceived by others, and they also serve to guide your clinical work. As a student in speech-language pathology, you will be using professional written communication across various practicum settings, and we hope that the general guidelines we have provided in prior chapters will serve you well. A book about professional communication, however, should discuss more than just the writing of reports. Communication takes place through several modalities and writing is only one of them. You will find that in every practicum setting, you will participate in verbal interactions with clients, family members, other professionals, and clinical supervisors. In most cases, these verbal interactions between people have an even greater impact on your clients, other professionals, and supervisors than your written reports. Verbal interactions are pivotal in the way you are perceived by others and central to how clients, families, professionals, and supervisors form an opinion about

your professionalism. Do not underestimate the importance of each verbal interaction you have with others because these exchanges have a significant impact in two critical areas. First, as stated above, verbal interactions are the primary determinant of another person's perception of you as a professional. Second, we use verbal interactions to gain information, counsel clients, provide information, and train others to participate in the treatment process. Although we could do all of these things in written communication, verbal communication generally facilitates a more engaging, open, and personal exchange of information between the clinician and others. Clients, family members, and other professionals have questions that must be answered by the clinician. In many cases, it is important to motivate clients and professionals to participate in the treatment program and motivate them to perform for greater progress in therapy. Perhaps more significantly, verbal communication adds the all-important human element to clinical practice. Face-to-face verbal interactions can often be the critical variable in success or failure of a treatment effort.

Your program may or may not have a course dedicated to the area of counseling or verbal communication. Regardless, it is an area in which you will need to refine your skills to best serve your clients. This chapter is designed to be an introduction to the foundations of effective and professional verbal communication and to review the varied aspects of interaction between you and those whom you serve. ASHA (2016) calls us to be responsible for this in its scope of practice document. This document states that SLPs are responsible for educating, guiding and supporting individuals with communication disorders and their caregivers by addressing "acceptance, adaptation, and decision making about communication, feeding and swallowing, and related disorders." This could include interactions involving emotions, thoughts, feelings, and behaviors resulting from the disorder. Please note that when we refer to the "client" in this chapter, we are being inclusive of any caregivers you may be speaking with as well, including parents, grandparents, or spouses of the clients.

Selected Critical Elements of Professional Verbal Communication

From examining the table of contents, you know that we present four separate chapters on professional verbal communication. This chapter focuses on communication with clients. The next three chapters address communication issues related to other professionals, individuals from diverse backgrounds, and clinical supervisors. There are, however, some critical elements that should be infused in professional verbal communication across all of these groups. Thus, while we discuss these variables here, you should remember that they should be part of all professional ver-

bal communication. There are many other characteristics that have been suggested over the years that contribute to effective interviewing and counseling. For example, Shipley (1997) lists the following: sensitivity, respect, empathy, objectivity, listening skills, motivation, and rapport. Many of these are subsumed under the five elements we discuss below. We have chosen only five variables because they are probably among the most important for beginning clinicians, and they relate to professional communication. Figure 10–1 illustrates five factors that should be present in all professional interactions, and we briefly discuss each of them in the following sections.

Show Respect

This component is something that should be part of any communication, whether professional or casual, but it is especially important for clinicians (Shipley, 1997). We want our clients, other professionals, and clinical supervisors to feel as if they are treated with respect for their infinite dignity and worth as human beings. Clients and families come to us for services to ameliorate a communication disorder that is having a negative impact on their lives. They may feel embarrassed and at a disadvantage when they need to come to a professional for help. We ask them for personal information about their problems, which again makes them feel vulnerable. These clients need to believe that the professional will treat them and the information they provide with dignity and respect. So how do we behave when we treat clients respectfully? First, it is common that at the beginning of the clinical relationship we refer to clients with a respectful term of address such as "Mr. Haynes" or "Mrs. Moran." This form of address connotes a professional relation-

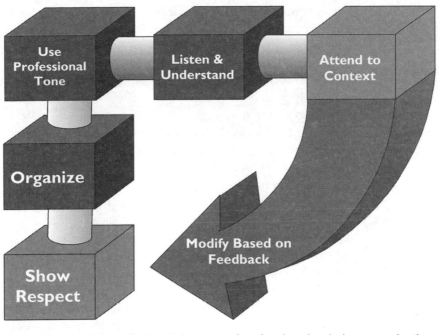

Figure 10–1. Selected critical elements of professional verbal communication.

ship and communicates respect for the client/family member. Obviously, after working with a family for a period of time, the person may say, "Please, call me Michelle." It is then appropriate to refer to the client/family member as he or she wishes, but we believe that it should be his or her call. Imagine yourself in a hospital after having a stroke. You have been deprived of all dignity and are in a vulnerable position. Then a stranger comes into your room and says, "How ya doin', Charlie?" This kind of familiarity from someone you have never met is not a respectful form of address. It is much more professional to say something like, "Hello, Mr. Haley, I'm Pearl Foy, a speech therapist. I understand you've had a stroke and are having some trouble talking." Just by using a term such as "Mr. Arnold," you have communicated respect for the patient. When dealing with other professionals it is always good to begin by using their title

(e.g., Dr. Abney) or calling them "Mr.," "Mrs.," or "Ms." You will find yourself working with psychologists, physicians, teachers, physical therapists, occupational therapists, and many other professionals who are consulting on your client. When you are at a staffing or introducing other professionals to family members, referring to them more formally is a sign of respect. As everyone gets to know each other, you will know when to refer to other professionals less formally. Regarding verbal communication with supervisors, it goes without saying that you want to strike a respectful posture with someone who is overseeing your practicum performance. Approaching clinical supervisors with consideration for their time and experience will help you develop the rapport necessary for a productive and healthy working relationship.

Respect for a person is also communicated nonverbally and by the physical environment in which you communicate. Your nonverbal behavior should suggest that you are genuinely interested in his or her concerns and take the interaction very seriously. A person may say all the "right" things, but body language such as fleeting eye contact, eye rolling, or appearing distracted with items can communicate disinterest. You should conduct professional communications in a comfortable, professional environment that protects client confidentiality and provides an opportunity for the person to express him- or herself without distractions. Making a person comfortable in a professional environment shows that you respect him or her as an individual and care about his or her concerns. Make an effort to monitor your nonverbal behaviors to ensure you are expressing your interest when speaking with others.

Organize

You will recall from Chapter 4 that we suggested one of the most important parts of writing reports is organization. Having organization to the information you provide makes the report follow a logical sequence and increases its intelligibility and ease of reading. It is exactly the same with professional verbal communication. No one wants to listen to a person who just rambles on in an unorganized stream of consciousness. A clinician has particular goals in mind when talking to clients, other professionals, or supervisors. For example, your goal might be to obtain specific kinds of information from a client or family member during a diagnostic interview. Obviously, it would help to have thought about the information you need and mentally prepare for the interview. Some clinicians make general notes to remind themselves to address specific areas of discussion in the diagnostic

interview. It is much better to be organized than to complete the interview and discover that you have not asked some important questions. Another example might be that you are asked to participate in a multidisciplinary staffing of your case with other professionals. Again, these professionals do not have time to listen to your rambling, and unorganized monologue. You should have your remarks outlined and any visual aids (e.g., handouts, treatment data) prepared prior to the staffing so that you can present a coherent description of your client. When talking with your clinical supervisor, it is always a good policy to organize your information prior to the meeting. If you are talking about treatment progress or you have questions for your supervisor, these can all be organized and discussed in a logical way rather than haphazardly. Thus, it is clear that verbal interactions with clients, other professionals, and supervisors are not mysterious and unpredictable. You should prepare for these meetings ahead of time by organizing what you will say and not merely winging it. You might have to do this on paper in the beginning, but with more experience you will be able to mentally organize your discourse.

Use Professional Tone

You will recall that we introduced the notion of *professional tone words* in Chapter 4. By using these words, clinicians make their reports sound professional, and it is no different in verbal communication. The key in both interactions is for the clinician to judge whether such terms would be appropriate for the person involved in the communication. For instance, if talking to a classroom teacher, a term such as *literacy* would probably be understood. Similarly, you might use the word *cognitive* when talking with a psychologist. On the other hand, if you were talking with a parent who had an eighth grade education, it would not be appropriate to use a term such as cognitive because the parent may have a misconception of the term. Thus, it is important to use professional tone words in verbal communication as much as possible, but you should always consider the background of the listener. Although you may want to impress them with jargon from your academic classes, you should make your best attempt to speak in language that they will be able to process and understand. You do not have to avoid using all jargon, but define any you use and attempt to provide an example to ensure comprehension. After hearing the client's concerns, you may need to adjust your typical presentation of results to accommodate a higher or lower level of education, or understanding. Just because someone has an advanced degree does not mean that he or she will automatically understand a complex description from you. When the use of professional tone words may result in confusion, it is important to simplify your language, in order to communicate effectively.

Listen and Understand

Professional verbal communication is a two-way street. You are not talking with clients/family members, professionals, and supervisors just to hear the sound of your own voice. Thus, it is important to be a good listener when engaging in professional verbal communication. Most counseling texts suggest that it is critical that we listen to others for both the *content* and the *affect* of what they are saying (Crowe, 1997). The notion of content refers to the actual words and information that the person is providing. For instance, if a parent says, "Jeremy said his first word at age 3," the content

would be the literal information provided by the mother. However, if the mother said the above utterance while a tear ran down her cheek and her voice broke in the middle of the sentence, this illustrates the affect or emotional tone of the utterance. Attending to both the content and affect of utterances in professional verbal interactions is very important. In the above illustration, we might want to engage the mother in further conversation about how she feels about her child's disorder. She may simply need to vent her concern and disappointment, or she may need a referral to a counselor if it seems like the feelings are affecting her life negatively. The point here is that we would not want to simply jot down that her child said his first word at age 3 and ignore the clear expression of emotion.

It is important to let your clients know that you empathize and care about them and what they are going through. Pindzola, Plexico, and Haynes (2016) offer the following suggestions for the occasions when clients express emotion:

- Avoid superficial statements of reassurance.
- Do not use terms or suggest consequences that will precipitate more stress for the client.
- Do not communicate any negative expectations regarding the outcome of therapy to the client.

Pindzola, Plexico, and Haynes (2016) additionally note that "the best antidote to fear and uncertainty is knowledge." (p. 47). This emphasizes the importance of your knowledge and ability to effectively relay the details to them regarding their disorder and treatment plan.

The same principle applies when working with other professionals. If you are trying to engage a classroom teacher to help with language stimulation for a preschool child and she says, "Sure, I'll help with the speech therapy; I don't have anything else to do," there is something more in that utterance than her willingness to assist in treatment. She is obviously feeling overwhelmed with her job responsibilities and viewed your suggestions as an unwelcome addition. If you attended to her emotional tone, you might say that you would be willing to come into the classroom and lead certain activities or assure the teacher that your suggestions can be implemented while she manages her regular routine.

The listening principle also applies to communicating with clinical supervisors. If you ask for therapy suggestions and your supervisor asks, "Have you reviewed in your class notes and looked up current research?" the real message is that you need to take more responsibility for coming up with ideas rather than being "spoon-fed" by your supervisor. Never underestimate the importance of not only *listening* but *seeking to understand* your partner's perspective in verbal communication.

Attend to Context

Every verbal communication takes place in a context. The idea of communicative context has several components to which a professional must attend. Specifically, we are referring to (a) whom you are talking to, (b) where you are talking, and (c) the feedback that you receive from your communication partner. First, you must consider the person to whom you are talking. This person possesses certain background knowledge based on experiences and education and represents a unique cultural history. Any verbal communication must take into account these "who" variables, whether you are speaking to clients/family members, other professionals, or your clinical supervisor. Let's say you are working with a Native American family from a lower socioeconomic level who has a child with a language disorder. You cannot assume that this family will inherently understand the nature, assessment, and treatment of child language disorders. Thus, your use of professional tone words will have to be reduced in favor of more "client-friendly" language. Several sources report that many cultures are not comfortable in revealing personal information to relative strangers (Battle, 1997; Roseberry-McKibbin, 1997). A good clinician will take this into account and perhaps postpone some of the more sensitive questioning until after a stronger relationship has been formed with the family. It is easy to see that appreciating the context of professional verbal communication is an important variable in interacting with clients. It is also significant when engaging with other professionals. For example, when you talk to a classroom teacher, you can assume background knowledge about the educational milieu and the types of problems typically seen in SLP and teacher collaborations. You can use "educational" vocabulary and even some vocabulary specific to SLP if you have worked with this teacher before. If the teacher is Hispanic, you want to make certain that you do not make any cultural gaffes in your conversation that might be offensive to a member of that ethnic group. Thus, the "who" of verbal communication partially defines how the conversation takes place.

The "where" of verbal communication also dictates the nature of a professional conversation. If you are talking in a hospital setting, it is appropriate to use medical terminology shared by physicians, nurses, OTs, and PTs. You can assume that a term such as *FIM score* will be understood by most people you are working with. But, even though you are in a hospital, you must also remember the "who" factor. If you are talking to a family member of a teenager with a head injury, the term *FIM score* will be meaningless, and you will have to modify your language to suit the listener. Similarly, when talking in an educational setting, you might assume that most teachers, special educators, and school psychologists share knowledge of certain terminology unless it is very discipline specific. At any rate, it is fine to throw around terms like *IEP* and *benchmark* with most educational personnel: just do not mention *diadochokinetic rate*.

Modify Based on Feedback

In any professional conversation with clients, professionals, and supervisors, there will be turn-taking and interchange of both verbal and nonverbal communication. Sometimes, even if you have been respectful, organized your thoughts, used professional terminology, listened to content/affect, and attended to context, there will be miscommunication and error. This is why a professional always examines the nonverbal and verbal feedback from a conversational partner. If you are explaining the assessment results to parents and they begin to look quizzically at you, it is time to rephrase your utterance so that it can be better understood. Parents or caregivers may be reluctant to ask you to repeat, so it is vital that you look for cues that they do or do not understand what you are saying. If you are explaining your test results/recommendations to a physician and he starts shaking his head, you will need to address any concerns that are present. Thus, it should be no surprise that professional verbal communication forms a feedback loop by which we constantly monitor our conversation and make changes to optimize communication. Ideally, we generate clear explanations on the initial attempt, but in cases where there is misunderstanding, we always have an opportunity to clarify.

The Value of Experience

As we stated earlier, the critical elements discussed above are a part of any professional verbal communication, whether it is to clients, professionals, or supervisors. As a beginning student in clinical practicum, you have no doubt admired the ability of your supervisors when talking with parents, family members, and other professionals. How did they get to be so confident and able to think on their feet? Well, like many other enterprises, it all gets easier with experience. As clinical supervisors, we understand that students typically feel underqualified and not equipped to evaluate, treat, and counsel adults as they are much younger than their clients or the caregivers they are interacting with. Be encouraged by the research of Haynes and Oratio (1978) on intervention effectiveness that found that adult clients value technical and interpersonal skills more than a clinician's age, gender, or race. Therefore, acting in a professional and pleasant manner is more influential to the client than the difference in age.

Most students feel completely inept when someone mentions the word "counseling." They frequently report that they do not feel competent in counseling another individual about anything, as the word *counseling* conjures up thoughts of delving into an individual's private life, using psychological lingo, and taking on the responsibility of someone else's problems. It is no wonder students shy away from any situation that might require they counsel their clients about their communication disorder. But, what we always tell students is that the way they become good at counseling is to listen to their clients and become as knowledgeable as possible about their clients' disorders. Then, students are able to approach their clients with sensitivity to their situations and counsel based on knowledge, backed by research and clinical practice, not on conjecture. Most people appreciate someone providing straightforward information in a gentle way about whatever it is they are dealing with. And unfortunately, many people are never told or understand exactly what their disorder is, what caused it, and what they can do. The competent, professional SLP attends to context to make sure he or she has done all he or she can to ensure the patient is educated and equipped to deal with the situation.

You will find that in the beginning of your practicum experience you will probably not be given assignments to talk with clients on your own. Instead, you will most likely observe sessions where your clinical supervisor leads the interview, parent training, or presentation of information at a staffing with other professionals. One reason why your opportunities for professional verbal communication will be limited at the beginning of practicum is that because it is a skill that does not come naturally to anyone. You first need to observe competent models of professional verbal communication from experienced clinicians. As you progress in clinical practicum, you will be trusted to take on more of the responsibilities of verbal communication with clients. By the time you are finishing graduate school, you will have seen many different styles of interaction with clients and their families. Ideally, you will be given opportunities to observe

your supervisors and allied professionals in a variety of counseling situations so you can learn from them. You will then find yourself incorporating the styles of various supervisors with your own personality, which will ultimately result in your own style of professional verbal communication. Before you graduate, you should have had the experience of a variety of types of verbal communication independently as you talk to clients, families, and other professionals.

Contexts of Verbal Communication With Clients and Families

There are at least six major contexts in which you will be using professional verbal communication with clients and families: (a) conducting a diagnostic interview with parents of a child client, (b) conducting a diagnostic interview with an adult client, (c) conducting a diagnostic interview with the family of an adult client, (d) conducting training sessions for patients and/or caregivers for a home treatment program, (e) discussing treatment progress with clients and/or their caregivers, and (f) counseling clients and/or their caregivers about treatment issues. Within each of the aforementioned situations, you will be interviewing, providing informational counseling, providing personal adjustment counseling, or a combination of these. It is impossible to do justice to the field of counseling in a couple of short chapters, so we will talk generically about the six aforementioned areas. We refer you to other sources for a more detailed treatment of interviewing and counseling (Crowe, 1997; Emerick, 1969; Pindzola, Plexico, & Haynes, 2016; Shipley, 1997). Although there are disorder-specific considerations for every type of communication impairment, there are also some general principles that can be applied to interviewing and counseling no matter what the disorder. We provide a brief sketch of some salient points from each area in the following sections.

In addition to the guidelines we have mentioned above, AIDET which was designed by the Studer Group, may also be used as a model for verbal communication. It is a tool to utilize when communicating with patients or clients to effectively provide pertinent information and education through a caring and compassionate customer service model. It was designed for direct patient interaction to promote comprehension of pertinent information and adherence to recommendations. Rubin (2014) reports that AIDET allows the provider to have a more human, authentic encounter with the patient. The components of AIDET are as follows:

A = Acknowledge: Address and acknowledge each person you interact with by name using appropriate nonverbal communication (eye contact).

I = Introduce: Introduce yourself and state your credentials.

D = Duration: Give an accurate estimation for how long the evaluation or treatment session will last, and when results or progress reports will be completed.

E = Explanation: Explain the purpose and the planned order of the session. Allow time for questions, and provide your contact information.

T = Thank you: Thank the patient and anyone accompanying the patient for their time and choosing you to evaluate or treat them. Thank any

family members or caregivers for their assistance in the treatment of the patient.

Informational Counseling

Informational counseling occurs when you educate the client with information regarding the type and severity of the disorder, communication strengths and weaknesses, and your recommendations. You will be given the opportunity to provide informational counseling during both evaluation and treatment sessions. Informational counseling requires preparation. In a situation in which you know you are about to evaluate or treat a patient with a specific disorder with which you are not familiar, take time to research the characteristics of the disorder so that you have a better understanding of the possible nature of the patient's concerns. Even if you are familiar with the disorder, it may be a good idea to again familiarize yourself with norms and/or typical development so you can provide concrete examples of what is expected with regard to your client's age, gender, background, and/or medical history. Sometimes clients have misconceptions about different aspects of evaluation, treatment, and prognosis and by researching the disorder prior to speaking with them, you will be able to dispel any myths they may believe.

After an evaluation or treatment session, it is appropriate to provide a summary to the client about your assessment of him or her, including strengths and weaknesses. Citing specific examples allows you to provide concrete and objective observations when discussing communication skills. Of course, it is always preferable to begin by describing strengths and then move to weaknesses.

When providing counseling after an evaluation session, the time in which you counsel a client or caregiver is dependent upon many variables. These include the type and severity of the disorder, type and extent of testing administered, client knowledge of deficits, and individual needs. Counseling after treatment sessions is usually more brief; however, this again varies on an individual basis and includes reference to performance and home program suggestions. Regardless of the situation, it is imperative that you allow the individual(s) a reasonable amount of time for information transfer and questions. You want to ensure the client has understood the vital pieces of information that you are wishing to communicate to maximize the effects of therapy.

Three Important Issues Common to All Diagnostic Interviews

We discuss some factors related to conducting diagnostic interviews with parents, family members, and adult clients in the next portions of this chapter. It is beyond the scope of the present text to provide detailed coverage of how to conduct interviews for every disorder seen by the SLP, but we will mention some important issues that are common to any diagnostic interview with any of the above groups.

The Interview Setting

Remember that one aspect of professionalism is the context in which clinical activity takes place. We want the interview room to be professional in appearance. This means it should be neat, clean, comfortable, and private. You must consider that the parents, client, or family members will be revealing personal information that should be kept confidential. This means that we do not perform a diagnostic interview in a waiting room or hallway. There should be some privacy provided for activities such as in an office or treatment/evaluation room.

Setting the Tone

A diagnostic interview is not simply a social chat. The interview is directed by the clinician, although the parents, client, or family members may not be aware that it is a directed conversation. It is up to the clinician to set the tone for the interview by telling the parents, client, or family members what will transpire (Matarazzo & Wiens, 1972; McQuire & Lorch, 1968). The box shows a brief example.

> Mr. and Mrs. Walsh, I'm pleased to meet both of you and your son, Brad. To begin, I want to let you know what will happen today during Brad's evaluation. I know that you have filled out the case history forms, and I appreciate you taking the time to do so. I was able to read those and I would like to clarify several things you mentioned in the paperwork to get more information that will help me as I do the evaluation. So, first we will talk about Brad, and then I will be giving him some tests and getting some samples of his communication. After I am finished with the assessment, I will meet with you again and let you know the preliminary findings and recommendations. At that time you might have questions that I can answer. It's better to save your specific questions for later on because I will be able to answer them more fully after observing Brad. Do you have any questions about what will happen today?

Notice how the clinician speaks formally, yet in a friendly manner. Note also that the clinician has sketched out how the evaluation will flow from obtaining information and assessing the child to providing information and making recommendations.

The Presenting Story

Most authorities on clinical interviewing suggest that clients come to the assessment with a "presenting story" that they have rehearsed prior to the actual meeting (Emerick, 1969). You have no doubt experienced this yourself as a patient going to a physician for diagnosis of a medical problem. On your way to the doctor you might think about the types of symptoms you have been experiencing and what you have done to help yourself. Some people even talk through this presenting story in their car while driving to the doctor's office. As a clinician, it is important to let the patient reveal the presenting story because it contains the patient's reason for coming into the clinic, his or her perception of the problem, and any misconceptions he or she might have regarding the situation. There are some ways to elicit the presenting story in the box.

> Adult client: I'd like to begin by having you tell me what led you to come to the clinic for an evaluation.
>
> Parent: So, what are your concerns with William's speech and language?
>
> Adult with precipitating medical event: I know you've filled out our paperwork, but can you describe your medical history and concerns for me?
>
> Spouse: Can you explain when you first became aware of differences in your husband's speech and what those are?

Notice how the clinician leaves it open-ended so that the respondents can describe in detail their concerns and issues. These can be followed up by questions from the clinician when information is not clear. It is always good to ask caregivers or clients for an example of behaviors they are concerned about. Sometimes clients, parents, or family members have misconceptions about their situation. We should always listen to these but not correct them at this point in the interview. Later, when we provide information about the evaluation we can clarify any misconceptions that exist. For example, see the box.

> *In the diagnostic interview* the mother says:
>
> William mispronounces everything and people can't understand him. I've got this Uncle Calvin who is slow and nobody could understand him either. We hope that William isn't, you know, like Calvin.
>
> *After the evaluation* the clinician says:
>
> Earlier you mentioned a concern that William might be misarticulating because of an intellectual disability. Most people with an intellectual disability who misarticulate have problems with vocabulary and sentence structure and show delays in many areas such as motor skills, social development, play, and activities of daily living. William has the language skills expected for his age and typical normal social, motor, and self-help skills. Based on formal testing and playing with him, I can tell you that he does not behave like a child with an intellectual disability. Research has shown that most children with articulation errors similar to William's are of average or above average intelligence. In his case, I feel the problem is confined to his articulation. He is not producing sounds, such as /th/, /l/, and /r/, and I feel that he could benefit from therapy to work on those.

There are three classical parts to a diagnostic interview, whether it is with parents, clients, or family members. According to Pindzola, Plexico, and Haynes (2016), the interview is designed to do three things *in this order*: (a) obtain information, (b) provide information, and (c) provide counseling if necessary. Let us briefly go over these three components of a diagnostic interview as illustrated with parents.

Diagnostic Interviews With Parents

One of the most important objectives of a diagnostic interview is to obtain information from the client/family. In some settings, the client may have completed a case history packet prior to arriving for the evaluation. In other cases, it may be completed upon arrival to the appointment. Regardless of whether you have information to review before, you will still conduct and interview. It is usually wise to focus on background information first to help you clarify for omissions and ambiguities in the case history. In many instances, responses on a case history form raise more questions than they answer. For instance, the parent might have indicated that the child takes a lot of medications, but neglected to mention what specific types of drugs are taken. You would want to follow up on this by saying, "In the case history you mentioned that your son takes several medications. Can you tell us what they are?" Sometimes parents will say something very general or ambiguous that you would like a specific example of, such as, "Joey has behavior problems." There are many types of behaviors that are typical in children (e.g., tantrums) and those that are of more concern (e.g., harmful self-stimulating behaviors). It is always good to solicit examples from parents if they have been ambiguous. You can see that there

can be many general issues to clarify in a diagnostic interview, and usually the initial part of the interview is spent addressing these background issues. But we are not done obtaining information yet. Some writers have characterized the diagnostic interview as a "funnel" in which we begin talking about general information and then focus more closely upon specific issues (Emerick, 1969; Stewart & Cash, 2010). Thus, we rarely go into a diagnostic evaluation of a child knowing nothing about the disorder of major concern to the family. Typically, we will have read case history forms that have been completed by the parents prior to the actual evaluation date or spoken with them over the phone. In most cases, the case history information will have a statement of the problem according to the parents, and this gives us a general guide to planning the evaluation. For instance, the parents might indicate that they are concerned about disfluencies, hoarseness, language development, or articulation errors. These statements of concern help us to focus the evaluation and the questions posed in the diagnostic interview. If the problem is hoarseness, you will want to ask questions about activities that could contribute to vocal abuse/misuse. You will also want to know how the vocal quality changes throughout the day, and if it had a sudden or gradual onset. There are many areas of questioning that are specific to each disorder of communication, and you should be prepared to ask them in an evaluation.

As you are selecting standardized and nonstandardized measures to use in the evaluation session, you should also be thinking about questions you would like to ask the parents when they come for the assessment. Organization has been a common thread winding through this text, and you can see that it is important in conducting a parent interview. Beginning clinicians should write down areas of concern in which more information is needed. We do not suggest writing down *specific questions,* because, as mentioned in a previous section, you do not know the parent's level of understanding. You could craft a specific question, and it might be too technical for some parents or not specific enough for others. Jotting down "areas" that you want to research is a more flexible approach. So, for example, if you have a concern about hearing loss and the parent has not addressed this in the case history, you should ask about hearing in the interview. The major point here is that you should never go into a parent interview unprepared. You should arrive at the interview with a legal pad that has specific issues written on it *in a logical sequence.* If you want to get more information on the biological foundations of communication, group your questions appropriately (e.g., hearing, motor skill, injuries, illnesses, medications). For example, do not skip from hearing to play to social friendships and then back to illnesses. Obviously, organization and planning of an interview can be done for any suspected area of concern in communication disorders whether it is language, phonology, fluency, or voice. You should look carefully at the case history information, class notes, and textbooks for specific background information for the type of communication disorder of concern to the parents. Before the evaluation, it is a good idea to show your proposed interview protocol to your supervisor. We guarantee you that the supervisor will be impressed with a student who has thought about and planned a clinical interaction with parents.

We need to mention an important thing about the conduct of a diagnostic interview. The clinician guides the conversation to gain an understanding of the client's history, current concerns, and personal goals. Interviews are not the same thing as a social chat that moves randomly from topic to topic. You should set the tone for the interview by telling the family how it will proceed. You can indicate that the first part of the conversation will be to get information from the family because, after all, they are the most knowledgeable about their particular situation and concern. Once the parents know that you want information to use in your assessment, they usually provide examples and answer your questions. Sometimes parents want to ask questions while you are obtaining information, such as, "When do you think Henry will talk?" A question like this is guaranteed to get you off track and at that point you do not have enough information to make an educated guess. You might say, "I'll be able to answer you better after the evaluation when I've had a chance to see how Henry does on our tests. We'll have plenty of time to go over everything, but right now I want to learn about what you have noticed at home." Once you have all the information you require, it is time to do the actual evaluation and gather data on the child's performance on standardized and nonstandardized tasks.

After the evaluation tasks, the parents will no doubt want to hear something about the results. No one wants to come to an evaluation and be told to go home without at least some preliminary information. Obviously, you will not have time to formally score all the standardized tests and transcribe/analyze a language sample on the day of the evaluation. You will, however, know some general pieces of information about the child's performance and will likely be able to recommend if therapy would be beneficial. Providing information can be conceived as having three parts. The first part of providing information is to summarize as many of the test results as you can, if only on a general level. Although you may not have scored a test, you will know that he missed a lot of items on certain sub-tests, or that he was able to complete other items without difficulty. You will know about language errors he made from a conversational sample. From your knowledge of normal communication development, you should know whether or not the child's performance is similar to other children at this age level. If you feel that the scores are borderline and you are not confident with your recommendations, you can postpone detailing your recommendations until the tests have been scored. After summarizing the general test results, you then move toward interpreting the test results and talking about prognosis. The parents need to know what it means when you say that he performed poorly on an articulation test, but his performance on language tests was normal. For example, parents may not know that phonological and linguistic disorders are often co-occurring, but in Henry's case, his main difficulty is with speech sounds. They also need to know that because he was stimulable, has normal hearing, has an interested family, and has no language problems, he has a good chance to perform well in therapy. After summarizing and interpreting the test results, you are ready to make recommendations. You might recommend treatment two times per week for 30 minutes to work on specific phonemes or phonological processes. The point here is that you have provided information in a systematic way, moving from test results to interpretation to recommendations. Again, organization is key to professional verbal communication. The box gives an example of providing information to parents of a child who was evaluated for a fluency disorder. Notice that the clinician summarizes the test findings, and then moves into interpretation and finally to recommendations. Note also that the clinician leaves time for the parents to ask questions.

The Results

Well, I've finished all of the testing and I'd like to tell you what I found. Michael did fine on all of the language and articulation tests I administered, so he seems to be developing sentence structure, vocabulary, comprehension of language, and speech sounds. He also has normal hearing according to the screening. I took a large conversational speech sample and I did notice various types of disfluencies in his speech. For example, he repeated whole words, phrases, parts of words, and some individual speech sounds when he talked. I also noticed some tense pauses in his speech where he abruptly stopped talking, breathing, and voicing. Another thing he did was to put what's called a filler in his speech, such as "uh" or "um." In addition, he showed some struggle behavior when he seemed to get stuck on a word.

Interpretation

So, Michael's language, hearing, and articulation results indicate he is where he should be for his age and I have no concern in those areas. In the area of fluency, it is important to note that most children Michael's age repeat words and sentences as part of normal development, and he has those kinds of repetitions in his speech. You mentioned earlier that you were concerned about the development of stuttering. Some of the things that suggest the possible development of chronic stuttering are things like repeating parts of words such as syllables, and repeating individual sounds such as "k-k-k-k-kite." Also, tense pauses and struggle behaviors are associated with the onset of stuttering in many children. You also mentioned in our earlier interview that Michael's uncle had a stuttering problem. If I look at all these things together, I feel that Michael is not merely producing normal developmental disfluency, but is exhibiting behaviors associated with chronic stuttering.

Recommendations and Prognosis

Because Michael is less than 4 years old, I feel he has a good chance to become more fluent with therapy. Usually, the earlier a stuttering disorder is diagnosed, the better the outcome with therapy. Also, because his language abilities are normal and you are motivated to work with him at home, the prognosis for improving his fluency is good. I would recommend that Michael come to therapy two times a week and that I work with you on some things that might help him be more fluent at home. Do you have any questions for me?

The final component of the diagnostic interview is providing personal adjustment counseling, if necessary. In the vast majority of cases, no counseling issues arise in the diagnostic session. Sometimes, parents will react emotionally if they are hearing for the first time that their child really has a communication disorder. Perhaps they have been holding on to the hope that their child has normal speech and language abilities and just wanted to have that notion confirmed. Another issue might be concern over finances and if they can afford to pay for treatment. Most universities have sliding fee scales, or the parents can be referred to the public school system where treatment is free of charge. The point here is that if a parent expresses a real concern, emotional or not, you cannot just send the parent home to ruminate about it. If there is something you can explain to ease the concern, you should do it. Again, in most cases this will not be necessary, but remember about the importance of listening for content and affect when speaking with your clients.

Diagnostic Interviews With Adult Clients and Their Family Members

You will notice that we have combined the next two areas of professional verbal communication with adult clients and families. Many of the same issues we raised in the previous section on diagnostic interviews with parents apply to these other groups as well. We are still conducting a professional interview, and there are goals of obtaining information, providing information, and counseling, as needed. There are some slight differences in working with adult clients and those who accompany them, such as a family member, friend, or paid caregiver. First, when interacting with parents, we are not asking the young child questions during the interview. The parents are the most reliable informants for younger children. For school-age children, however, it is critical to actively involve them in the interview to get the most comprehensive information. In the case of adult clients, however, many can speak for themselves and should be allowed to do so unless they are unable. For example, a client who has had a stroke and cannot speak would not be able to provide information during the evaluation. In that case, interviewing a family member is a reasonable method of obtaining this information. We must always be careful, however, to maintain the dignity and respect of the client. We do not want to talk about the client as if he or she is not there. If possible, it is always good to involve the client in the interview, if for no other reason than to confirm what the family member has said. Some clinicians ask questions first of the patient, and then turn to the family member if the patient is unable to respond. Then you can ask the patient if that information is correct, or make a comment related to the new information. Even if you do not ask a question, you can let the patient know where you are going with the interview. For example, you might say, "I'd like to learn a little about the work that you did with the government. Is it all right if I ask your wife to tell me about that?" Again, you are still trying to obtain information from the client or family member, just as you would do when talking to parents.

In most cases, adult clients are fully capable of speaking for themselves. Adults who stutter or have minor language problems, phonological disorders, or a voice disorder can give you information directly during the diagnostic interview. Even if they are able to answer your questions, it is also beneficial to get feedback from caregivers or family members. For all adult clients, you must organize your questioning in a logical sequence for the disorder area that is of concern to the client, just as we illustrated in the previous section on the parent interview. Obviously, with an adult client, your questions will revolve around vocational and daily obligations, rather than their performance in school and achievement of developmental milestones. The order of the diagnostic interview, however, does not change. First you obtain information, and then you administer various diagnostic tests. After testing, you provide information about test results/interpretation and make recommendations. If the client has major questions or concerns that require brief counseling, you provide it as needed. Margolis (2004) compiled the following suggestions based on numerous research studies to effectively communicate diagnostic recommendations and results.

Methods of Maximizing Retention

- When giving instructions, use concrete terms. "Say each word on this list, emphasizing the /f/ sound and ask your child to repeat" is more effective than, "Here is something to practice at home."
- Use language that is easy to understand.
- Provide the most important information first (the primacy effect), which is often a recommendation.
- Emphasize key points of recommendations or other information.
- Inform the patient of the order in which you will be presenting information. For example, "We are going to go over recommendations, then we will talk about your child's language abilities (diagnosis), then we will discuss test results, then we will talk about the plan of treatment and what you can do at home." Be sure to solicit questions before moving on to the next category.
- State the most important information more than once.
- Do not overwhelm them with information. Provide only the information they need at that time.
- Seek to understand the patient's goal for the evaluation and their perspective of the problem.
- Provide written, graphical, and pictorial materials to supplement verbal explanations.

Conducting Training Sessions for Developing a Home Treatment Program

In most treatment approaches that seek to improve speech and language, it is desirable to develop a home program to facilitate the generalization of communication skills learned in the clinic to other environments. Usually, the success of home programs hinges on the amount of direct training provided to the family and client and the clinician's ability to communicate what is to be done. Therefore, for a program to be successful, there must be some type of organization and clarity in presenting the information to parents or clients. Paul (2006) outlines many parent programs that take a structured approach to language training for generalization to the home environment. In other words, for a home program to succeed, the parents or family members must be specifically trained to implement the generalization activities. You are not establishing a home program when you walk the client down the hall after therapy and suggest the client does a little of this and a little of that. Such suggestions, although not harmful, are not likely to be implemented correctly, or implemented at all, for that matter. On the other hand, if you use the last 10 minutes of your treatment session to invite the parent or family member into the therapy room and actually show him or her what to do and let him or her try it, that is a different story. Then you can take the opportunity to give feedback pertaining to the way he or she is performing the technique and provide reinforcement and suggestions. Our point here is that home programs can enhance generalization, but home programs are not as effective without specific training. This training is done through the use of professional verbal communication.

At times, we wonder why clients do not use strategies or information we give them for use outside the therapy room. It may result from them not understanding what we said or being too embarrassed to ask questions to clarify. Alternatively, they could be doing what they thought we said when that was not the suggestion at all. Fourie (2009) provides guidance for this process and notes that adults with acquired communication disorders appreciate the SLP providing knowledge to them in terms that they can understand and providing practical and concrete suggestions.

The first step in training a parent or family member is to organize your training regime. There is that word again: *organization*. You must put some thought into what you want to establish, the procedure to be used in training, and the most effective way to communicate this to the parent or family member. This is applicable to any type of training whether it is directed at language stimulation, reduction of vocal abuse, responding to disfluencies, or generalizing gains made in correct production of misarticulated phonemes. One important thing should be clear from the outset. We want the home program to involve fairly simple, straightforward, and manageable tasks that can easily fit into the daily routine. The parent should not be trained to do complex treatment tasks that are difficult to learn and do reliably. The general progression of such training has several components, no matter what the disorder area targeted. First, the clinician must tell the parent/family member about the general goals of the home program. If it is a child language case, it might be the use of recasting at home to facilitate generalization. Specifically, let's talk about a child who substitutes him/he and her/she. This child might say, "Her is my sister." We are working on the correct use of pronouns in clinical sessions, but we want to involve the parents in a home program to facilitate generalization. Much research has shown that recasting has been effective in training language across many different groups of children and a variety of language structures (Nelson, Camarata, Welsh, Butkovsky, & Camarata, 1996). So, in this first step, we need to tell the parents that there is research that supports the use of recasting in language training, and this is a technique that is fairly easy to learn and implement during daily interactions in the home environment. The clinician might define recasting as restating the child's incorrect utterance in a correct manner. For example, if the child says, "Her is my sister," the parent should say, "Yes, she is your sister." Recasts can easily be woven into conversations, and they do not require the child to imitate or correct the utterance. They serve the purpose of giving the child a correct model of a sentence that the child has produced incorrectly.

After outlining the technique that you want the parents to use, you move on to step two. In the second step of parent training, you actually demonstrate the technique with the child in the therapy room with the parent watching. In this way, the parent can see the procedure in action and it is not simply an abstraction that was talked about in step one. After several demonstrations, you move on to step three. In the third step, the parent is encouraged to try the technique with the child and the clinician provides feedback about effective use of the technique and anything that might be changed to make it more productive. In the fourth step, the parent is asked about situations in the home environment where recasting might be used. For instance, the parent might say that a lot of conversations with the child occur in the car when running errands and going to various sports practice events. This is a good time to have conversation and use recasts. Finally, the parent is asked to make some mental notes about the child's correct production of the target language structure. That is, we want the parent to notice if the child is beginning to use the correct forms more often.

It is clear that training parents/family members to do any type of home program is done by professional verbal communication. We explain, model, monitor, and charge the parent/family member with the responsibility of implementing the technique. This applies to everything from articulation disorders to vocal abuse to stuttering. The key is that the training is organized and professionally done by the clinician.

Discussing Treatment Progress With Clients and Families

It is the responsibility of any competent clinician to provide feedback to clients about how they are making progress in treatment. Ideally, this is done by presenting behavioral data showing that performance has changed over time. Again, this is accomplished using professional verbal communication. Certainly, you can give copies of treatment reports to clients/family members, but in most cases such reports are written in terms that are more appropriate for SLPs and other professionals. It is always a good policy to sit down with clients/family members and take stock of progress or lack thereof. In the university clinic, for example, the end of the semester is a good time to have such a conference. In the medical setting, you may be called upon for a brief report whenever a family member's visit overlaps with your therapy session.

As in any professional verbal communication, organization is again a central issue. You should not sit down with clients to casually discuss clinical progress without adequate preparation. Some obvious components of that preparation would be the data gathered throughout the semester, and in most cases it is good to display the data on a chart or graph. If the graph shows an increase in performance of treatment targets or a decrease in errors, most parents are satisfied that they are getting their money's worth. When explaining treatment progress, it is a good idea to recap the goals targeted in therapy and how they relate to the data presented. Another part of a treatment progress conference is to talk about the next set of goals that will be targeted in the next semester and ask for feedback from the parent or client. Although we all would like to make progress in treatment, there are cases in which the conference will demonstrate a decided lack of progress. If the graph is not moving away from baseline levels, then the discussion with the parents might focus on variables that need to be changed in order for progress to occur. For instance, a child who comes to treatment once a week for 30 minutes and is not making progress might need to try coming twice a week in order to have a positive response. Again, the data you present will support your suggestion. Do not forget to solicit client feedback in these progress conferences. Are there things they are especially pleased with regarding the treatment? Are there aspects of the therapy they do not understand? Do they have any concerns or issues they would like to raise? All of this is done using professional verbal communication, and it is a critical component of a good clinical relationship with clients or families.

Counseling Clients and Families About Treatment Issues

On a realistic level, counseling in a clinical relationship is designed to solve problems and/or deal with feelings related to the treatment regime. Many types of problems may be associated with treatment such as irregular attendance to therapy sessions, lack of progress, unrealistic expectations on the part of the client/family, feelings of hostility or discouragement related to the treatment, lack of motivation, explaining changes in the treatment approach, transition to another service provider, or refer-ral to a professional from a related discipline (e.g., psychology). Actually, the issues listed above might very well account for most of the counseling efforts in treatment encountered by students in clinical practicum, but there are certainly others we have not raised. Even though you may not have a long history with the client, you will have to deal with the day-to-day occurrences that happen in the therapeutic relationship. Thus, it is the goal of this section to provide a *general* view of the process of communicating about counseling issues rather than an all-encompassing set of guidelines. For more detailed coverage of counseling, we direct you to other sources (Crowe, 1997; Shipley, 1997).

Figure 10–2 shows a very basic process of identifying and dealing with treatment issues using professional verbal communication. This is fundamentally "problem solving"; however, you will see that confronting problems in clinical work often leads to talking about feelings and perceptions that are more sensitive than a simple social conversation. Thus, the approach we are taking to counseling is a series of steps for addressing problems that arise with clients in your practicum experience. We briefly discuss each step below, and guess what? Organization is a major factor in counseling, just as in every other aspect of professional verbal and written communication.

The first step in counseling about treatment issues is to identify the problem. In some cases, the client will be the person who identifies an issue of concern. For example, after a treatment session one day, a client might express dissatisfaction with the amount of progress being made in therapy. Your first reaction might be to act defensive about such a comment, and you might feel bad about your performance as a clinician. A positive aspect of this comment is that the client has brought it out into the open

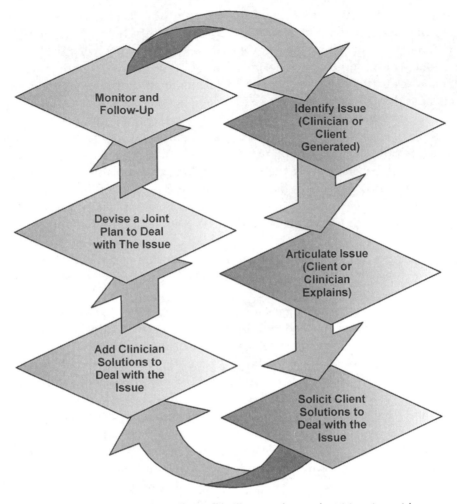

Figure 10–2. Counseling clients/family members about treatment issues.

and has not internalized it and simply sabotaged the treatment by not trying or failing to attend therapy sessions. A good clinician simply cannot let this comment go by and not deal with it. Thus, we have a situation in which a client has identified an issue (dissatisfaction with treatment progress) and the clinician must find a way to explore the problem and suggest solutions. The second step in this process is to obtain the client's perception of the problem. Typically, the clinician can act as a facilitator to gain more insight into the issue. For instance, the cli-

nician might say, "Let's talk about this for a while. Tell me some specific things that you are not satisfied with in our treatment approach or your progress. Then we can make some adjustments to the therapy or talk about your progress and how we can improve our approach." This opens up a "can of worms," but you can clearly see that allowing a client to go through the motions in treatment sessions while harboring such feelings is not productive. In some cases, there is simply a misunderstanding of the goals or unrealistic expectations on the part of the client. These can easily be dealt with by counseling the client on the difficulty of treatment and providing examples of the range of progress made by many clients working on the same type of communication disorder.

Sometimes there is a specific issue that is bothering the client. For example, a client who stutters might be frustrated with clinical exercises involving easy onset and slowed speech rate because no generalization to daily situations is seen where the stuttering still occurs. Again, this can be dealt with by further explanation of the techniques, or more realistic situations can be integrated into the treatment in which the techniques can be used to facilitate fluency in everyday communication. Whatever the situation, it is always better to address it than ignore it.

After identifying the issue and articulating it, the focus should be on potential solutions to the problem. If you have not learned this already as part of your life, solutions are generally better when arrived at jointly by the people experiencing the problem. It is a wise clinician who solicits client solutions to a problem and then suggests some additional solutions to the mix. So we ask the client, "What do you think we can do to make better progress?" In some cases the client may say that more treatment sessions are needed. In other cases, the client may feel the clinician is not being aggressive enough in treatment. Other cases may want some different aspects added to the treatment approach. The next step is for the clinician to add possible solutions to those that the client has provided. Be sure to reinforce the client's suggestions if they are reasonable. "I really like your suggestion of using more realistic situations in therapy. Actually, I've got a whole file of real-life activities that we can arrange in order of difficulty and start using next week if you like."

So both the client and clinician have made positive suggestions for the treatment approach and the next step is to agree on a joint plan of action. If the client likes some of the ideas that were generated in joint discussion, the plan needs to be formalized. "Okay, it sounds like we are in agreement about the problem and some potential things to try in order to solve it. I'll bring my list of activities on Monday and we can prioritize them so we can work toward you being able to use your techniques in more realistic situations." Now, it might occur to you that the client may not be ready to produce fluent speech in more difficult situations. What if the person fails at the new activities? This is not all bad, because it may just be the dose of reality the client needed to justify more work on easy onset and slower rate in the clinic. All the counseling in the world may not make the client feel good about boring clinical activities, but experiencing difficulty on higher level tasks might bring home the realization that a bit more practice on the easy onset and slower rate is not such a dreadful idea after all. If the client is successful at more difficult tasks, it merely shows what a good clinician you are, because you have responded to client suggestions that allowed faster treatment progress. If the client is not successful, again you have been responsive to concerns, but you were correct in your initial judgment of client abilities, and it is now clear why you started at that level.

The final step in the process is to monitor how the plan has worked. After trying out the plan agreed upon by the client and clinician, it is always a good idea to take stock of how things are going. "Well, we've tried some more realistic activities and you seem to be responding well according to our data on your disfluencies. How do you feel about your progress in therapy now?" This gives you an opportunity to attain closure on a problem that has been solved, and it also opens the door to making adjustment in the treatment that will fine-tune the approach.

Remember that we said the counseling issue might be raised by either the client or the clinician. For instance, the clinician may be concerned about the client's attendance, the inconsistent use of practice outside the clinic, or the lack of motivation. Any of these issues can and should be raised if they are on the clinician's mind. "We have you scheduled for therapy three times a week, and yet you are only coming one or two times. I'm afraid that this might be having an impact on your progress. There are a lot of reasons why people come inconsistently ranging from scheduling to money to transportation to motivation. So, tell me about why you are having trouble getting here and maybe we can come up with a plan to make things better." Again, you could just let it slide and not say anything, but you are not dealing with the underlying problem. Opening the door to discussing such issues is much better than ignoring them and hypothesizing all sorts of reasons that may not be true. Whoever raises the issue, client or clinician, the important thing is that the concern receives your attention. These concerns are dealt with exclusively using professional verbal communication as you identify issues, articulate them, solicit joint solutions, devise a cooperative plan, and monitor the plan to determine if it was or was not successful.

Personal Adjustment Counseling

Fourie (2009) notes that SLPs need to be ready not only to treat the communication impairment itself, but also the issue of the impact of the communication disor-

der on the client. This type of counseling encompasses being available to assist your client in coping with the information you have provided. Dependent upon your setting, you may encounter a person who has experienced a life change such as a stroke, diagnosis of head and neck cancer, or the recent diagnosis of a child with autism or cerebral palsy. The client may be experiencing grief, anxiety, shock, frustration, or anger, and you should be ready to listen when the client shares his or her concerns. Ignoring the client's concerns or changing the subject will communicate to your client that you are either disinterested or do not approve of what the client is feeling. Kaderavek, Laux, and Mills (2004) found that the clinical counseling relationship significantly influences positive client outcomes. Therefore, if you do not effectively address your client's needs and concerns, progress may be hindered with regard to therapy goals.

We would like to be clear at the outset: Counseling a client is serious business that takes years of training and experience to perform well. Just to give you some insight, Crowe (1997) discusses some of the following counseling opportunities that arise in SLP, depending on the client's age and type of disorder: (a) feelings of anxiety, grief, guilt, isolation, and anger; (b) denial of the problem; (c) dealing with a guarded prognosis; (d) self-concept; (e) cultural barriers; and (f) inaccurate perceptions and nonproductive attitudes. Shipley (1997) raises the specter of clients who are paranoid, overprotective, talk too much, are depressed, and may even contemplate suicide due to the changes in their lives after a stroke, laryngectomy, or degenerative neurological disease. Obviously, we do not expect students in training to delve into the psyches of their clients and deal with these major emotional and life issues. In some cases, even the experienced SLP must refer such seriously involved clients to professional counselors or psychotherapists. Most of the time, we can deal with clients having a bad day by just being human, listening to them, and demonstrating that we understand their feelings. No one who is feeling depressed wants another person to deny the validity of his or her feelings and pretend that everything is all sweetness and light. Clients who become frustrated and depressed about their abilities after a stroke might say, "I used to be able to do woodworking in my workshop, but since the stroke, I can't use my tools. That was my favorite hobby and now I can't do it." A validation of their concern would be an appropriate response, such as, "I know how much you loved woodworking and it must be very frustrating not to be able to do that anymore." Remember the content and affect concept. In most cases, for practicum students, there are more basic issues to deal with that involve professional verbal communication. If serious counseling issues come up, the student needs to (a) recognize the issue, (b) address it if it is a fairly simple and straightforward problem, and (c) alert the clinical supervisor if the problem seems beyond his or her ability to deal with. It is always better to err on the side of caution rather than dabble in issues you are not equipped to handle. Your own experience will be a guide as well. For example, once you have counseled parents on children's behavior problems with the help of your supervisor, you should feel some confidence in addressing similar issues with a new case. But, if your client with a laryngectomy says she has no friends and does not want to live, you probably need to get some help from your supervisor.

It is tempting to want to focus specifically on your client's speech and language issues, but you must learn to view the client as a whole person, with needs in areas outside their communication skills. The focus should be on the client and his or her needs, rather than on you and the agenda you have for the evaluation or treatment session. According to Kaderavek, Laux, and Mills (2004), "This process includes learning to tolerate silence during the client-clinician interaction, to reflect client emotions, and to clarify clients' self-perceptions" (p. 154). Luterman (2001) noted that "clients' self-discovery and self-actualization is best accomplished by listening instead of prescribing." Moments of silence should not be feared but welcomed as a means of encouraging the client to continue speaking and to process information that you have communicated to the client.

During treatment sessions, you may be forced to modify your plans based on the client's demeanor and level of motivation for that day. Therefore, it is pertinent that you take your lead from the client, and that you listen to the client so you know how best to provide information and emotional support. Hackney and Cormier (1994) noted that the use of minimal encouragers, such as "mmm-hmm," "yes," or "I see," communicated the attention and approval of the clinician. Another aspect to consider is what you are communicating to the client through your nonverbal behavior. Appropriate facial expressions, deliberate head nodding, and a relaxed and slightly forward body position are regarded as indicating favorable affect and encouraging the client to speak more (Kaderavek et al., 2004; Mehrabian, 1972; Shipley, 1997).

At the same time, you do not want to abandon therapy goals while the patient spends the entire session lamenting his or her troubles. Davis (2000), as cited in Fourie (2011, p. 58) gives advice for this. "On some days a patient may just want to talk, and a clinician may want to be sympathetic to the client's desire. However, the clinician has to make a judgment as to whether listening for a while is necessary for achieving successful stimulation on that day. The patient may need to vent, which should clear the air to resume treatment. In general, the clinician needs to manage valuable treatment time by gently steering the patient into planned activities." When listening and then responding to your clients' concerns, you can reassure them by remaining calm and collected while problem solving with them regarding the issues related to their communication disorder.

The degree to which you serve as counselor varies according to the individual, his or her disorder, cultural background, issues stemming from his or her disorder, or other life issues. It is vital for you as a professional to be ready to provide all types of counseling, as necessary for you to establish and maintain rapport with your client and/ or their families. That being said, it may become apparent during your sessions that your patient could benefit from formal psychological services. It is your responsibility to address this need with your client and provide recommendations regarding possible resources and referrals. As cited in Atkins (2007, p. 5), ASHA stated that SLPs should "support their client's emotional and psychological concerns as they relate to the communication disorder." It may be necessary to provide support in dealing with issues resulting from a client's communication disorder, but it is not within the SLP's scope of practice to engage in formal psychotherapy. Although you may feel that you know exactly what course of action the client should take, avoid trying to solve the client's problems. Counseling a client is quite different than counseling a personal friend, and this requires awareness on your part to respond in an appropriate manner.

Scenario 1

You are in the middle of a diagnostic session with a client who has recently had a stroke. Your supervisor has told you to administer the *Boston Diagnostic Aphasia Examination*, and emphasized how important it is to complete the test for treatment planning purposes. After completing only two subtests, your client suddenly begins to tell you how upset he is about his inability to drive, and he begins crying and states that he does not want to be a burden on his family. What do you do? Although you may be tempted to avoid the issue and continue with the test, it is necessary and appropriate to stop and listen to what he is saying. Allow him to express his concerns, using empathy and good listening skills. If your client is given the opportunity to express his emotions in a nonjudgmental and supporting environment, you are on your way to establishing trust and rapport. More than likely, you will be able to continue the assessment with your client less distracted and able to persevere with genuine effort. If the concern is related to an allied professional (in this case an Occupational Therapist), make that referral, or if necessary, refer to a counselor or psychologist.

Scenario 2

You have been working with a 2-year-old client for approximately 5 weeks. Your client is nonverbal and demonstrating behaviors that are consistent with Autism Spectrum Disorder, although he has not been diagnosed. At this time, he has been diagnosed with a receptive and expressive language delay, and possibly Pervasive Developmental Disorder (PDD). One day, your supervisor is away from the clinic at a conference, and your client is avoiding eye contact and exhibiting various types of self-stimulating behavior. The parent comes up to you after the session and asks, "Do you think my child has Autism?" What do you do? Even though you are not qualified to make this diagnosis, you are able to say to the parent, "I understand your concerns, and based on what I've learned in my classes, I have seen some behaviors that are common in children on the spectrum. Next week, my supervisor will be back, and I will arrange for her to discuss this with you prior to the session. It may be necessary for us to make a referral for your son to be evaluated by another professional who could do additional testing prior to a diagnosis."

This chapter aimed to illustrate some basic principles of professional verbal communication with clients and families. As a student in clinical practicum, you will do far more communicating verbally than on paper with your clients and family members. This verbal communication is a platform by which you obtain information, provide information, and deal with problems that arise in the course of your clinical relationship. Always remember to be respectful, organized, professional in your language, a good listener, and attend to the context of communication so that your utterances will be appropriate in terms of the environment and the client's knowledge base and culture.

If you remember these things when communicating verbally, you will be perceived as a professional. Also, know that problems are bound to arise in any clinical relationship. It is always best to deal with such issues earlier rather than later. Whether the client raises the issue or you must bring up a sensitive problem, these concerns can be dealt with in a systematic way using professional verbal communication. The problem must be identified and discussed. A joint plan of action must be devised using input from both clinician and client. Finally, a mechanism to monitor whether or not the problem has been solved must be put into place. Throughout your career, you will be called upon to provide counseling to persons of all ages with various cultural, educational, cognitive, and socioeconomic backgrounds. Remember that it is your job to respectfully provide them with clear, pertinent, and accurate information related to their communication disorder and specific strategies to increase their communication skills in their daily activities. Also, it is not your job as clinician to "cheer them up," but to empathize with them and then assist them in identifying possible solutions. Such problem solving is always a challenge, but it is a natural part of clinical responsibility, interaction, and ultimately success.

11

Interacting With Other Professionals

In the beginning of your clinical practicum experience you will probably have little opportunity to directly interact with other professionals. This is because initial practicum assignments are typically in the university clinic. Usually, such clinics are staffed solely by speech-language pathologists and audiologists, unless the clinic operates in tandem with other departments on campus such as special education, psychology, or health professions. Although such models exist on university campuses, they are not the norm. As you progress in your practicum experience, you will find yourself interacting with more professionals from other disciplines when you are assigned to rehabilitation centers, hospitals, schools, or long-term care facilities. Even in the beginning, however, you might have the opportunity to collaborate with other professionals on a case you are involved in within the university clinic. For example, you may be working with a child who has a language/phonological disorder. It is possible that this child is attending public school and is receiving treatment from the school speech-language pathologist (SLP). This child will also have a classroom teacher and may be receiving other services from a specialist in learning disabilities. Thus, even though your work is confined to the university clinic, you might come in contact with these other professionals for a variety of reasons. First, you might be interested to know about the Individualized Education Program (IEP) goals that your client is working on in the public schools. To find this out, you have to contact the school SLP either in person, by telephone, or by e-mail to obtain the relevant information. A second reason is to determine how your approach at the university could make the best contribution to the child's overall treatment regimen by coordinating your goals with those of the school personnel. For instance, they might be working on literacy skills and grammar, but have little time to work on phonology and pragmatics. The university program could plan to target a variety of goals so that some are not ignored or duplicated across settings. A third reason to contact the school professionals is to determine how the work you are doing with the child in the university clinic is generalizing to the school environment. You may want to visit the school and observe your client's communication in the academic setting. During this visit, you will no doubt come in contact with professionals who work in the school system. A final reason to contact the school personnel is to determine what curricular materials might be used in your therapy to result in maximum generalization. Most authorities in school-age language disorders suggest that treatment activities incorporate some academic material such as grade- or subject-specific vocabulary and discussion topics so that the child can receive an academic payoff in addition to the communicative gains.

Depending on the type of case, there may be other professionals involved in treating your client simultaneously. Some campuses, for instance, have programs for children with autism, and the child may be attending a program in the department of special education or psychology. In this circumstance, you might be doing your treatment either in the university clinic or in these other departments. Either way, you are in a position to interact with other professionals. Thus, you can see that interaction with other professionals can take place even when you are operating in the sheltered environment of the university clinic. As we said above, such interactions will only increase in your practicum experiences that take you to other settings throughout graduate school and in future employment.

In Chapter 10, we outlined several critical elements that should be part of professional verbal communication with clients and families. These elements were showing respect, being organized, using a professional tone, listening/understanding, and attending to the communicative context. All of these elements, crucial to interacting with clients/families, are just as important when communicating with other professionals. We give several examples of how these factors apply to our conversations with professionals in this chapter. We just wanted to bring them back to a conscious level for the present chapter. It is assumed that you will attend to these critical elements of interaction in all your communications with professionals from other disciplines.

Contexts of Professional Verbal Communication With Other Professionals

There are at least four contexts in which you will be likely to interact with professionals from other disciplines: (a) consultations, (b) staffings/meetings, (c) collaboration, and (d) solving problems in informal daily interactions. We discuss each of these below to give you a flavor for how they unfold.

Consultations

In most instances, the purpose of a consultation is to access additional information or a different perspective on your client. The time spent seeking information about your client from another professional allows you to obtain valuable discipline-specific information that will assist you in your treatment program. We mentioned above a situation in which you might want to obtain information about the school curriculum and/or goals that the school SLP is targeting in treatment. In most cases, for this to be done effectively, a face-to-face meeting or a phone call is necessary since it is difficult to cover all the information using written communication. Typically, persons elaborate more verbally, and speaking with someone results in a more comprehensive picture of the client. However, due to the demands of the schedules of allied professionals, e-mail may be the most convenient choice.

When working with a child who has been diagnosed with autism, you might have questions about how to manage behavior problems that occur during treatment. In your search for answers, you might ask the psychologist who is treating your client to consult on the case. For the consultation, you could meet with the psychologist to discuss your concerns either in his or her office or in the speech and hearing clinic. During the meeting, you should ask the psychologist to provide suggestions for effectively managing behavioral issues. As you progress in practicum to other work settings, it is not unusual to ask other professionals such as physical therapists, occupational therapists, nurses, or physicians for a "consult" on a patient you are both treating.

There is also the possibility that you are seeing a patient who is not receiving services from another professional and you feel that the patient might benefit from an assessment and/or treatment. If you question the need for a formal referral, you can ask for input from a colleague who works in your organization or one employed outside your facility, if needed. In these cases, you can describe your concerns about the client without disclosing any confidential information. Formal referrals for evaluation are done when you are confident that the client needs a comprehensive evaluation. These are done on a fee basis and often need doctor's orders or other administrative paperwork to occur. As mentioned in Chapter 3, it is crucial to obtain a signed release of information from the client/parent before involving another professional in order to protect client confidentiality. Never underestimate the importance of obtaining a release of information before *any* consultation is done. Assuming we have permission, we might find the SLP asking the occupational therapist or physical therapist about positioning issues when working with a client who has a motoric disorder. Because these other professionals are working with the client on activities of daily living, they are usually more than happy to give suggestions about positioning the client for activities involving the SLP. Similarly, other professionals will ask the SLP about the communicative status of a patient with whom they are both working and how to interact effectively. Such informal consults are part of working together as a rehabilitation team and should be done frequently to promote the best care of your client.

Consultations are a professional courtesy and when asking another professional for a consultation, it is important to remember that you are requesting a favor. Thus, you can see why showing respect, organizing your request, talking professionally, listening carefully, and attending to context are critical. The box illustrates an example with a psychologist.

Telephone Contact

Hello Dr. Jarvis, this is Madeline Smith and I'm a speech-language pathology student working in the university speech and hearing clinic. I recently spoke with Mrs. Caldwell, and she gave me permission to contact you about her son, Kevin. I'm working with Kevin on producing single words to communicate his needs and wants. Kevin is exhibiting some behaviors that I am having difficulty managing in his sessions. I know that you were able to assess Kevin recently and was wondering if it would be possible to set up a short meeting with you? I would like to get your input on how to effectively manage Kevin's behavior and increase his attention span during our sessions.

The Meeting

Thank you so much for taking the time to talk with me about Kevin. I would greatly appreciate any insight you might provide so I can treat his language disorder more

> effectively. One of his treatment goals is to use a word to request items to play with during therapy. Frequently, when I ask Kevin what toy he would like to play with, he responds by hitting and spitting. Right now, I'm dealing with this by telling him "No" when he does these behaviors, but it doesn't seem to reduce their occurrence. Do you have any suggestions?

Notice how the clinician called to set up the appointment to see if the psychologist was willing to consult. Also, note that the clinician got right to the point, by explaining her goals and concerns. You can see that organization was important in obtaining this consultation. There was preparation in terms of locating the correct telephone number, making an appointment, selecting an example of the behavior that was of concern, and telling the psychologist how the behaviors are currently being handled. The goals of the meeting are to communicate your questions clearly and obtain specific answers in order to provide optimal treatment for your client. A meeting with another professional can save you a lot of time and energy in the long run. After the meeting, it should go without saying that the clinician thanks the psychologist for the consult. It is always a nice touch to give feedback to the other professional, especially if his or her suggestion has been implemented and it was effective. Everyone likes to hear that his or her advice was followed and helped the situation. Also, it never hurts to let the other professional know that "if there is ever anything I can do for you on a case in the future please let me know." Usually, professionals involved with a common patient are very interested in what your goals are for the client and how you are targeting them. The box gives an example in a school system of consulting with a teacher.

Initial Contact in the Hallway

Hi, Mrs. Alsheri, I was wondering if I could get some advice about one of your students. Because you are his teacher and know how he responds, I'd like your input on incorporating some classroom material into his language goals. If you are willing, I'd be happy to come to your classroom at a convenient time for you to get your opinion on what I'm doing to incorporate the curriculum into his therapy.

The Meeting

Thank you so much for taking the time to meet with me. I'd like to talk about Stephan. I've brought the materials I'm using with him and I wanted to show you how we are trying to incorporate American government into our language goals. You can see that I've made an organizational chart we can use when we discuss how the government works to make laws. I was wondering if there are any other strategies you are teaching in the classroom that I can help him practice in our sessions.

Notice how the clinician approaches the teacher in a respectful manner and requests a convenient time to talk about the student. At the meeting, the clinician is well prepared, organized, and asks specific questions about how to use classroom work in treatment.

Consultation is an important component of the relationship between various disciplines. As your career progresses, you should be prepared to both request consultation from and provide consultation to other professionals. Consultations may involve a scheduled meting as shown in the above examples or simply a brief conversation with the other professional. If you have only a question or two or a quick piece of information to share, a meeting may be unnecessary, such as in the following example.

Consult in Office With Physical Therapist

Good morning, Stuart. Do you have a minute to talk about Mr. Williams? I know you said in the team conference that he was having difficulty following your directions while you were treating him. I was able to complete my assessment yesterday, and he has significant auditory comprehension deficits due to aphasia and a hearing impairment. Can I make some suggestions that might make it easier for you to communicate with him? I know it is noisy in the therapy gym where you are treating him, so finding a space away from other patients will help reduce some of the competing background noise. Before you give him instructions, make sure he is looking at you and give short, concrete instructions, using gestures when possible. If you find any other strategies that you feel help him, please let me know and I will do the same.

Note that the SLP was respectful of the physical therapist's time by asking if it was convenient for him and keeping the conversation succinct. Specific, concrete suggestions were provided and were applicable for the physical therapist's setting. The SLP concluded by inviting the physical therapist to add his input, which communicates the acknowledgement of the value of his feedback of the client's communication skills as well. Verbal communication is the major vehicle for consultation, and for success to occur, it must be done in a professional manner.

Staffings and Meetings

In many work settings there is often the opportunity to "staff" a case that has common interest to a variety of professionals.

Staffings usually focus on sharing multidisciplinary assessment or performance information from a variety of professionals. The two environments where staffings are most common are medical facilities and school systems. In some university clinics, students are asked to meet for the purpose of discussing their cases as part of a "grand rounds" experience or merely a case presentation. Such experiences in the university clinic give the beginning student a chance to organize and cogently present information on a client to faculty and peers in the training program. Presumably, it prepares these students for presentations they might have to make in the future. For example, in school systems there are IEP meetings and other opportunities to discuss the progress of students receiving therapy. In medical facilities, staffings are common and are attended by representatives of all health professions involved with the patient. Often, these staffings are weekly, or even daily, especially in facilities where the patient is staying for a limited time frame.

The conduct of a staffing is much like any meeting where there is an agenda. The purpose of the staffing is for all of the professionals who work with the patient to update the team regarding progress toward goals and any difficulties that may have arisen since the last meeting. Typically, one professional (and it could be from any discipline) directs the meeting. This person is often called the case manager and will facilitate the agenda of a staffing in which treatment progress is discussed by the medical or educational team. In some facilities the staffing concerns many patients, each of whom must be talked about by all relevant professionals. In these types of staffings, time is of the essence and each professional is allotted only a few minutes to report on the patient's progress. Thus, you will only have a short period of time to let the other professionals know how a particular patient is progressing toward goals. This is one reason why FIM scores are commonly used in medical facilities. It does not take long to report "Mr. Jackson has moved from a level 5 to a level 6 for language comprehension." In other settings, however, the meeting or staffing concerns only a single client. For instance, there are clinics that provide in-depth multidisciplinary evaluations, and the purpose of the staffing is for each professional to provide detailed information on his or her assessment and finally to engage in a discussion of the combined results to arrive at treatment recommendations. Obviously, in this type of meeting you will have the floor for a longer period of time and go into significantly more detail. In some medical settings, complex cases are reviewed in detail with lengthy presentations by different professionals and a group discussion of recommendations.

If you are scheduled to participate in a staffing of your client next week, there are several things you should do in preparation. First, you should find out the nature of the staffing in terms of time allotted to each participant. It makes a great deal of difference if you have to prepare a 5-minute presentation or a 30-minute case summary. For our purposes, let's assume that you are scheduled to talk for 15 minutes about your case and the progress he has made in treatment over the last 3 months. If you have read this textbook thus far, you already know that merely showing up at the staffing with no preparation is not an option. Organization and preparation give you the opportunity to make a successful and informative presentation that benefits your client. Lack of preparation will result in a poor to mediocre presentation that will not reflect positively on you or the facility you represent.

After finding out the type of meeting you will be attending, you should assemble all of your data on the client so you can determine the information that will be the most relevant. In this particular case, you are charged with presenting information on the client's progress over a 3-month period. Thus, you probably will want to spend most of your presentation time on this topic rather than an extensive reiteration of the client's case history or the client's status 6 months ago. Although it is certainly acceptable to mention some historical information and intake data, your focus should be on the past 3 months. In many cases the same professionals sitting around the table will have attended a meeting on this same client 3 months ago when you talked about earlier therapy progress. In this case, they are familiar with background information and the client's baseline performance. So how do you prepare yourself to present the treatment progress over the last 3 months? A logical place to start is to mention all of the goals you were working on during that period. This can be followed by the presentation of treatment data and description of performance on each goal, perhaps supported by graphs or handouts. SLPs can share communication and cognitive strategies for other professionals to encourage the client to use throughout the day in order to generalize targeted skills and maximize communication with others. The final portion of your presentation might focus on goals that have been accomplished and the establishment of new goals to be targeted in the next 3 months. Notice that the presentation is organized, focused, and packaged to fit into the time allotted. It is also important to remember that you must take into account your audience when you are presenting information at a staffing. Although you can use professional terms that cross disciplines, any concepts unique to the SLP should be explained in easy-to-understand language to avoid confusion.

If you are not the first one to present, it is often useful to refer to the presentations of others to validate points you need to make in your summary. For example, if the occupational therapist reports that the patient has difficulty paying attention while completing activities of daily living, you might say, "Just as OT indicated, I have also noticed attention difficulties during my language treatment tasks." It not only shows that you are listening, but it validates the observation of someone else on the team and helps to consolidate information on the patient. Just as in consultations, staffings provide you the opportunity to share helpful strategies you are using with the client to improve areas of difficulties, such as attention.

Staffings are not just serial reports by representatives of varied disciplines. Subsequent to individual reports, there is usually discussion centered on trying to integrate discipline-specific information and modify future goals based on client progress. Often, the discussion turns to problem solving in difficult cases. An important thing to remember is that you are part of a team that must reach some sort of consensus. You must strike a balance between raising issues and solutions you feel are important and allowing others to do the same. Staffings in which professionals provide no input and those in which a person dominates the group are equally unproductive. Remember, the welfare of the client is the most important consideration in any staffing.

Staffings are an important part of working as an SLP. They should never be taken lightly because you are not only representing yourself and your facility, but the entire profession of speech-language pathology as well. Staffings are accomplished almost exclusively with verbal communication among professionals, so students should take advantage of every opportunity to watch how these unfold.

Collaboration

For years, SLPs have cooperated with professionals from other disciplines in what has become known as a *consultative model* or *collaborative model* of treatment. In these models, professionals from varied disciplines work together to treat a particular client. Haynes, Moran, and Pindzola (2006) outline collaborative models in terms of interdisciplinary, multidisciplinary, and transdisciplinary approaches to therapy. Each of these approaches involves members of various disciplines, but the interaction among the professions is quite different. In multidisciplinary approaches, for example, each profession sees the client separately and there is very little cross-disciplinary planning. There are separate and discipline-specific evaluations, goals, treatments, billing, and parent/family conferences. As mentioned above, a staffing may occur at some point, but it is usually discipline specific. A multidisciplinary staffing would consist of each discipline presenting goals for the client and the progress achieved.

Interdisciplinary approaches are usually a bit more collaborative in that various professionals might, at least informally, discuss the client and try to cooperate on goals. There are still separate treatment sessions for each discipline, but perhaps the biggest difference between multidisciplinary and interdisciplinary cooperation is that there is a little more joint goal setting and communication among the professionals.

In transdisciplinary collaboration, there is the most communication and cooperation among professionals. The psychologist may actually work on communication goals at the same time as behavioral objectives. The SLP might incorporate motor skills into the treatment sessions for communication goals. The classroom teacher might assist in communication goals in the context of the classroom. There is much literature on consultative models used in assessment and treatment, and it is beyond the scope of this text to elaborate on this research (Damico, 1987; Ferguson, 1991; Frassinelli, Superior, & Meyers, 1983; Fujiki & Brinton, 1984; Magnotta, 1991; Marvin, 1987; Montgomery, 1992; Moore-Brown, 1991).

It is important, however, for beginning practicum students to see that, depending on where you are doing therapy, you may experience a variety of types of treatment approaches. Each of these different models of treatment involves changes in the types of professional verbal interactions you will have with other disciplines. These range from very little communication and collaboration (multidisciplinary) to frequent and close communication and collaboration (transdisciplinary). You should be able to see at this point that in multidisciplinary approaches, you are pretty much on your own in terms of assessing, developing goals, providing treatment, and evaluating treatment progress. On the other hand, in a transdisciplinary model you will have to communicate and cooperate with all the other disciplines involved to assess, develop goals, provide treatment, and evaluate treatment outcomes. In such a model you might be doing your therapy in the classroom environment instead of a therapy room. You may also be reinforcing academic goals in your therapy and behavioral goals suggested by the psychologist. In transdisciplinary models, everything is negotiated among the professionals involved, and this is all done by means of verbal communica-

tion. Some guidelines for conducting collaboration with other professionals were presented by Haynes et al. (2006). We briefly paraphrase some of those points below.

Administrative matters include the following:

- When using a collaborative model, it should not be an informal process, but should be formalized at a meeting. The group of professionals should assemble and discuss the collaborative treatment approach for the client.
- After the discussion, someone on the team should be designated to write down the treatment approach and everyone's responsibilities so that this information can be included in the client's folder.

Attitudinal variables include the following:

- You should listen attentively to other professionals on the team and "show respect and consideration for the other team members' expertise, questions, opinions, decisions, concerns, or goals involving the client" (Haynes et al., 2006, p. 33).
- You should assume a positive attitude and be sure to reinforce other professionals for their good ideas.
- Make sure you have studied the client's folder and note any concerns that you want to address with the group.

The following are considerations when conducting meetings:

- Make sure that each professional has an opportunity to provide input.
- Use "situational leadership" in which the professional with the most expertise on an issue (e.g., psychologist, SLP, teacher, PT, OT) takes the lead in discussing the topic.

- It is important for team members not to come to the meeting with a preconceived idea of what will be done. This is not working as a team; it is assuming that you have the best idea and it should be implemented. These meetings are not designed for one person to convince the other professionals to approach the treatment according to a single perspective or plan. The group should discuss the tactics for dealing with the problem and devise a joint approach to accomplishing goals.
- Do not use too much discipline-specific jargon. This interferes with communication and is a subtle way of putting other team members in a subservient position of having to ask for clarification.
- The team should devise specific goals for the client, assign responsibilities for targeting them, and discuss how they will be evaluated and who will assess the progress toward the goals.
- As mentioned above, this should be formalized in a report following the meeting and included in the client's folder.

No doubt, you can see that collaborating with other disciplines takes time, planning, preparation, and professional verbal communication. While it takes effort to collaborate with others, both the client and the professionals benefit from the process.

Solving Problems in Informal Daily Interactions

In any relationship, including professional ones, there is always the possibility that interpersonal difficulties can arise. Although there are many areas in which interpersonal problems can occur, in our experience there are three major categories likely to be encountered by beginning students in clinical practicum: (a) mistakes, (b) misunderstanding/miscommunication, and (c) crossing discipline boundaries.

Making Mistakes

The first area of interpersonal difficulty involves making errors or mistakes in assessment, treatment, or clinical reporting. First, *everyone* makes mistakes at some point. You tend to make fewer mistakes with experience, so students in training are a "high-risk" population. Hopefully, your clinical supervisor can help you avoid major errors, but there are always some that slip through. One thing is certain: once you make an error, you should learn from that experience and not let it happen again. That is one difference between you and your clinical supervisor: The supervisor has had the opportunity to make errors over a long period of time and learn from those mistakes, and you are only beginning. What kinds of mistakes are we talking about? Obviously, you will make many mistakes in writing clinical reports, but those are between you and your supervisor. Those errors never make it out into the world for others to see. In verbal communication, however, you do not have the luxury of a rough draft and soliciting comments from your supervisor. Thus, those verbal errors are not as easily retrievable. For example, you might have given information at a staffing that was incorrect or misinterpreted. In this case, the other professionals on the team may not know that the scores you presented were wrong and take them at face value. Obviously, if you said the child scored in the 80th percentile on a language test, but it was really the

8th percentile, this represents a major discrepancy. In cases like this, it is important for you to admit your mistake as soon as possible and explain the true nature of the situation. Everyone makes mistakes; it is only when you do not acknowledge them or try to hide them that you get into trouble. Other professionals will respect you more for finding and admitting your error than if you did not report it at all. Imagine your embarrassment, if after working with the client for a long time some other professional finds a discrepancy and brings it to the attention of the group at the next staffing.

The same principle applies to treatment objectives. Let's say you recommended in a staffing that certain goals should be a priority for language intervention. After working with the client for a while, you realize that the goals you set were far too ambitious and difficult for the client and you need to select other goals that are more realistic. Other professionals will respect your clinical decision to change your goals after considering the client's performance.

Because we know that this area presents a learning curve for students in training, there are several proactive principles to keep in mind. First, you should check and double-check your work so that mistakes can be found and corrected before you communicate them verbally. You cannot do a good job of professional verbal communication if you are relying on inaccurate data. A second principle to keep in mind is to think about what you are planning to say before you open your mouth. Make sure it is based on accurate data and not speculation. Make sure you think about saying it as professionally as possible. If you are not sure, ask someone such as a mentor or supervisor who is willing to provide helpful advice. Remember, once you say something, it is out there in the environment. You cannot, as they say, "un-ring a bell."

Misunderstandings and Miscommunications

Another area of potential difficulty with other professionals is misunderstanding and miscommunication. This is not just limited to the use of technical, discipline-specific language; it can arise from many directions. The box shows some examples.

OT: Mr. Liu's family told me that you said he will not ever be able to feed himself. Feeding is one of our major goals, and I don't appreciate you telling the family he won't be able to do it.

(Actually, you only said to the family that Mr. Smith was having some difficulty with feeding himself, among other aspects of activities of daily living, including communication. You never said anything about prognosis or the future. This was a misunderstanding and exaggeration by the family that was passed on to the OT.)

Teacher: Jalen's parents told me at our conference last week that you said I wasn't doing a very good job of teaching him how to read. I don't like it when other people undermine what I'm trying to do in the classroom.

(Actually, you said to the parents that children with language impairment often have difficulty learning to read and might need some extra help from time to time. The parents interpreted this as the teacher not doing her job.)

SLP: Richard seems to be missing many of the cognitive attainments that are associated with language development.

Psychologist: SLPs are not qualified to assess intelligence; that is the job of the psychologist!

(Actually, you were only talking about certain cognitive play behaviors such as object permanence, means-end, symbolic play, and functional use of objects that are related to language development. You were not making judgments about his overall intelligence.)

School Principal: My teachers tell me that you are complaining about the room that you use for speech therapy. You need to know that we have space limitations here and everyone cannot have exactly the type of room they want.

(Actually, you did say to two teachers that, because you were assigned to work in the cafeteria on the stage behind the curtain, it was a bit noisy for some of the distractible students, especially when the custodial and kitchen staff were setting up for lunchtime.)

All of these situations were the product of misinterpretation or miscommunication among various professionals. In each of the instances, the result was one professional being upset because of something someone thought you had said or done. These situations are unavoidable due to human nature. People do not always render an accurate report of what others have said, and the result is misunderstanding. If these situations are not dealt with, it could result in damaging the professional relationship you have with people from other disciplines. As a result, it could lead to unsuccessful collaborations and ultimately hurt the clients we are trying to serve.

In all of these situations, the antidote is effective professional verbal communication. First, it is important to notice the fact that a person is upset over something she feels you have done. This may be communicated directly as in the above examples, or indirectly by nonverbal cues or reports from others. Again, it is important to look at both content and affect of what some-

one says to you. Once you perceive there might be a problem, you need to address it as soon as possible. When a situation is ignored, negative feelings can incubate, and a strain may be placed on the relationship. Therefore, it is vital to communicate to the other person that you understand what he or she is feeling.

In the first example above, you might say something like, "That kind of statement is very upsetting to me, and I know it must be to you as well. I know that you are working on feeding, and if the family wants to know about prognosis, they need to talk to you. Let me see if I can clarify what happened. The family was expressing some frustration about how little progress he was making. I recall telling the family that Mr. Liu had difficulty in many areas including communication, walking, feeding, and cognitive issues, and that it is a challenge to have so many things to work on at the same time. I don't know how they translated that into a negative prognosis for feeding, but I'm sorry for the misunderstanding. I would never make statements to a family about something in your field. You are the expert on those issues, and I value your judgment and our working relationship." Notice several things. First, the response validates the person's feelings about being upset. Second, the response tries to address the concern directly and put it in the context of what actually occurred. Finally, the tone of the response gave respect to the other professional's expertise and role in treating feeding issues. It might have been easy for the OT to just ignore the comments from the family, but if that happened, resentment could build toward the SLP and a relationship could be affected or impacted. It is always good to confront such issues head on. If there is a logical explanation or misunderstanding, most people will accept this as a resolution to their concern. If, on the other hand, you have made a mistake or a misstatement or have actually said an unprofessional remark, you need to apologize for it and move on. It is easy to misspeak or to make a statement in confidence to someone you trust, only to have it revealed at a later time. It is a good policy to never say anything that you do not want another person to hear.

A final area of possible communication difficulty with other professionals revolves around crossing discipline boundaries. Professionals are known to exhibit a certain amount of "turfism," meaning that they perceive specific areas and procedures to be part of their field and no one else's. If another professional "steps on their turf," they become defensive and upset. Because communication sciences and disorders overlap with many other disciplines, it is not unusual for us to inadvertently step over a line or two as we interact with other professionals. Think about it. We work with teachers, nurses, physicians, psychologists, administrators, OTs, PTs, social workers, and other SLPs. Many of the issues we experience are the same as those dealt with by other professions. In the case of treating a child with behavior problems, the professional addresses these issues at the same time he or she is trying to accomplish the goals in his or her field of expertise. Thus, the teacher must minimize behavior problems during the teaching of science. Similarly, the psychologist must curtail behaviors while teaching the student how to

cope with them, and the SLP must learn to manage them while teaching language and pragmatics to the student. At a staffing, it would be easy for the SLP to describe "the best way" to handle behavior problems, but you can see that this risks stepping on the boundaries of the psychologist. Diplomacy is very important in professional verbal communication. It is better to say, "I'm not the authority on how to best deal with these behaviors, but here is what I have been doing in language therapy. I would be interested to get some input from Dr. Wilson (psychologist) on this issue." In this example, you admit that behavior problems occur frequently in your treatment sessions, but you also defer to the psychologist in terms of soliciting suggestions from the person who may be more qualified in the area of concern. In many work settings, disturbances in professional relationships can often be traced back to one person stepping on another's turf. Be wary of this next time you are tempted to give advice on topics that are only ancillary to your area of expertise.

This chapter focused on professional verbal communication with people from other disciplines, which can be the source of much joy or strife. Although verbal communication is often the cause of interpersonal difficulties, it is also the solution. Keep the channels of communication open, and you will be well on your way to becoming a professional who is admired, respected, and valued.

12

Interacting With Individuals From Diverse Backgrounds

Introduction

It is estimated that one in every 10 Americans, across all ages, races, and genders, has experienced or lived with some type of communication disorder (including speech, language, and hearing disorders), and that nearly 6 million children under the age of 18 have a speech or language disorder (National Institute on Deafness and Other Communication Disorders [NIDCD], 2016). With an estimated 322 million people in the United States (U.S. Census Bureau, Population Estimates, 2016), this encompasses an incredibly large group of people. Interestingly, the U.S. Census also shows that the number of foreign-born residents is projected to rise from 31 million in 2000 to 48 million in 2025. The Hispanic population alone (the largest minority group) is projected to triple by mid-century, and Asian Pacific Americans, the fastest growing ethnic group, includes more than 60 separate groups. In addition, the latest Census data indicate that almost 14% of U.S. residents do not speak English, creating a challenging clinical environment for speech-language pathologists (SLPs) and audiologists.

Across most service-related disciplines, the issue of multicultural diversity is a much publicized, and much criticized topic. Much publicized, because of the significant demographic changes that are taking place in the United States, and much criticized because clinical educators and students agree that most health professional programs fall short in preparing students to work with culturally diverse individuals. And in the field of speech-language pathology, this is no exception. In an article on its website, the American Speech-Language-Hearing Association addressed the issue directly. According to the article, "ASHA has targeted increasing the cultural competence of speech-language pathologists (SLPs) and audiologists as a strategic objective in its pathway to excellence" (Lemke & Dublinske, 2008). As a result, there have been a number of initiatives on the part of ASHA to promote cultural diversity. This is mostly due to clinicians and educators continuing to report concerns regarding the provision of services to culturally and linguistically diverse individuals.

Cultural Competence and the SLP

What is cultural competence? In short, it is developing an awareness and understanding of how individuals interact in the world based on the philosophy and beliefs of the culture to which they belong. Students in speech-language pathology will have numerous opportunities to meet and form relationships with people from a myriad of backgrounds and across the life span. Becoming culturally competent will ensure that you are well prepared to assist any person with a communication disorder, regardless of the person's background, or to what degree it is similar or different from yours. There has been a great deal of research on multicultural issues and how they affect the client/clinician relationship. It is sufficient to say that we do not cover the depth and breadth of that information in this chapter. What we hope to do, however, is to give you an idea of how you can begin to start moving toward cross-cultural competence, even as a beginning clinician.

Stewart and Gonzalez (2002), in an article on the role of SLP graduate programs in preparing student clinicians to serve a diverse population, identified multicultural training goals for SLPs that include increasing diversity of SLPs, increasing the quantity and quality of research, and improving academic and clinical preparation. It is to this end that we felt it necessary to introduce the speech-language pathology student to multicultural issues regarding the clinical practicum experience in order to facilitate student growth into a competent clinician.

There is no question that students in the field of speech-language pathology will be faced with understanding how to interact with and quite possibly counsel individuals from diverse backgrounds. One way to improve your skills as a clinician is to develop cultural sensitivity, or a willingness to learn about and address the needs of *every* patient. Working with someone from a culture that differs from yours naturally creates an opportunity for you to establish rapport and communicate effectively with this person, simply due to the fact that you are aware of their cultural differences. As a result, you are probably more sensitive to cultural norms and mores, and take great care in making sure you honor those. Most people are keenly aware when someone looks, talks, or acts differently than people from their own culture and background. You may even become aware that "your way" of communicating with someone may not be appropriate, effective, or even understood. It is always important to put yourself in someone else's shoes, as the saying goes, in order to truly establish a positive, successful relationship. As stated by Battle (2002), when counseling individuals from diverse cultural backgrounds, it is important to adhere to a basic set of guidelines, which can be best explained as a three-step process:

1. Counseling should begin during the initial evaluation so that the client and his or her family members or caregivers understand what will take place. The clinician will want to be aware of cultural beliefs about the necessity of the intervention process.

2. The clinician should always make sure the client and/or family members understand the diagnosis, prognosis, and any therapy techniques that may not be straightforward. Clinicians should remember to observe rules for cultural interaction (verbal, nonverbal, and social).

3. The clinician should be aware of personal adjustments of the clients and significant others as an ongoing part

of the treatment process. It is important that the clinician explore the possible significance of cultural mores and rules with regard to cultural identity and/or generational factors (age and maturity).

Even though a clinician may have a desire and a willingness to learn about others, it is impossible to learn everything about different cultures. Table 12–1 is a guide to various social interaction styles of the largest minority groups living in the United States in comparison to Anglo-European or American culture. It is our hope that this information will be beneficial to the SLP in following the guidelines mentioned above.

According to ASHA, "Culture can be viewed broadly as the socially constructed and learned ways of believing that identify groups of people, and verbal, as well as nonverbal communication behaviors readily identify cultural groups" (2004). Additionally, culture has been more specifically defined as integrated patterns of human behavior that include the language, thoughts, customs, beliefs, values, and institutions of racial, ethnic, religious, or social groups. Cultural competence is the development of a set of behaviors, attitudes, and policies that come together in a system, agency, or among professionals and that enable effective work in cross-cultural situations. According to the Office of Minority Health, a division of the U.S. Department of Health and Human Services, "cultural competence is important because health care services that are respectful of and responsive to the health beliefs, practices and cultural and linguistic needs of diverse patients can help bring about positive health outcomes."

Let's examine how cultural competence ties in with delivery of speech-language pathology services, whether in the university clinic, public school, or medical set-

tings. When the SLP enters into a clinical or therapeutic relationship with clients and their families, caregivers, or significant others, there may be some preconceived ideas about the individual. This could be based on the patient's name, age, referral source, place of birth, or even diagnosis. It is natural for people to make assumptions about someone they have never met based on certain factors. Unfortunately, these assumptions are often prejudiced, discriminatory, or simply inaccurate. A good clinician does not allow stereotypes, judgments, or preconceived notions to affect his or her ability to thoroughly assess and outline an effective treatment plan for clients who may be from a different culture than their own. A good clinician looks at the therapeutic relationship as one that both parties (the client and the SLP) can learn and optimally benefit from.

The Therapeutic Cycle

According to Johnson (2012), it is important for clinicians to realize that various aspects of culture such as customs, learning styles, beliefs/values, and social interaction style may influence the cycle of activities in a therapeutic relationship. The cycle of activities, or the cycle of the therapeutic relationship, as described by Stockman, Boult, and Robinson (2004), is defined as follows:

- Referring: providing access to clinical services
- Scheduling: selecting the time for a patient to receive clinical services
- Gathering information: obtaining patients' pertinent background information
- Assessing: determining the nature of a patient's communication disorder

Table 12–1. Greetings and Customs for Interacting Among Various Racial and Ethnic Groups

Ethnic or Racial Group	Greetings	Customs for Interaction or Visiting
Anglo-European American	• Warm, firm handshakes with direct eye contact are expected • An arm's length is considered one's personal space that should not be violated • Males usually shake hands with males, although there are no rules against women shaking hands with men or young persons shaking hands with the elderly • Turn-taking during conversation is important • Personal topics, personal self-disclosure, and controversial issues are avoided	• Punctuality is expected • Direct, face-to-face communication is expected • Personal opinions are expressed openly
African American	• Address by surnames and title (e.g., Mr., Mrs., Miss, etc.) unless permission is granted to use first names	• Avoid telling the family that they are touchy about racial issues • Avoid racial jokes even about one's own culture • Avoid stereotyping African American families • Do not talk with coworkers about personal matters • Do not judge family function by socioeconomic status
Asian American	• Address by surname • Avoid prolonged eye contact • Avoid physical touching • Greet family members from oldest to youngest Handshaking • Only males shake hands • Youngsters do not shake hands with elders	• Avoid personal questions during initial contact • Remove shoes when entering the home • Sit with feet flat on the floor and hands folded in your lap • Accept food or drink if offered • Demonstrate emotional restraint

Table 12–1. *continued*

Ethnic or Racial Group	Greetings	Customs for Interaction or Visiting
Latin American	• Speak to husband before the wife if both are present • Use a calm tone of voice • Initial "small talk" is important for establishing rapport • Provide background about what can be expected in future interactions	• Respect cultural artifacts/rituals and their importance to the family • Do not rush or be impatient, which shows disrespect • Do not be too direct • Build interpersonal relationships • Sit with good posture • Avoid the term *illegal alien*; use the term *undocumented immigrant* instead
Middle-Eastern American	• Personal space or social distance is shorter than for Anglo-European Americans • Men may kiss other men on the cheek upon greeting • Women may exchange hugs and/or kisses upon greeting • Avoid direct or assertive communication	• Remove shoes when entering the home unless family does not • Accept food and/or drink if offered and partake in the hospitality • Do not sit with your back to an adult who is present • Sit with legs up or crossed in front • Stand when new guests arrive, particularly the elderly
Native American	• Initial "small talk" is important for establishing rapport • Provide background about what can be expected in future interaction	• May not answer knocks at the door or doorbell • Ask whether an appointment is convenient (scheduling a time may not be as good) • Ask family where they would like you to sit • Family members may come and go from the home • Confidential topics may best be handled in the office • Accept food and/or drink and partake in the hospitality • In rural areas, unscheduled visits should be signaled by a honking of a car horn

Source: Based on Lynch, E. W., & Hanson, M. J. (1997). *Developing Cross-Cultural Competence: A Guide for Working With Children and Their Families* (2nd ed.). Baltimore, MD: Brookes.

■ Recommending: advising and/or counseling the patient about potential treatment plans

■ Treating: ameliorating or lessening the impact of the patient's communication disorder

■ Discharging: terminating the therapeutic relationship

In this section, we examine each aspect of the cycle in a little more detail:

1. *Referring:* Even with specific programs in place such as Child Find, Early Intervention, Medicaid screenings, and well-baby visits to pediatricians, cultural and linguistic barriers often prevent young children from getting the help they need. Parents who do not speak English may not understand the purpose of the screenings, the importance of follow-up testing, or the need for referrals to other professionals. This is where an interpreter can make the difference in a child or an adult receiving the intervention necessary to improve his or her quality of life.

2. *Scheduling:* A referral usually results in scheduling an appointment with a speech-language pathologist, whether at a private clinic, public school, or university clinic. Again, parents from culturally diverse backgrounds may not follow through if they do not know the reason for the appointment. They may also be apprehensive about returning calls to unfamiliar, English-speaking individuals. According to Johnson (2012), "Families of culturally and linguistically diverse backgrounds may value punctuality differently than mainstream culture and may be late to their scheduled appointments. Western cultures value punctuality more than

Latino, Native American and African American cultures do (p. 57)". She adds that clinicians should exercise positive regard and consider that tardiness to appointments may be due to cultural differences rather than a lack of respect.

3. *Gathering information:* Obtaining information for the patient's case history may be difficult, especially if the patient or caregiver does not speak English well. Having an interpreter to assist in filling out this form, or even having a form written in Spanish or another language would be beneficial. Be advised, however, that individuals from some cultures are reluctant to share personal information with professionals; therefore, this may also be a barrier to obtaining an accurate case history.

4. *Assessing:* This may be difficult for a myriad of reasons; some of which are quite obvious. Patients (children or adults) will not be able to respond appropriately to an assessment tool if they do not know what to do. In this situation, use of an interpreter is highly recommended. If an interpreter is not available, family members may be able to assist with communication. In some clinics, Spanish versions of commonly used speech and language assessments are available. The speech-language pathologist uses every resource possible to obtain valid assessment results. Quite often, an interpreter can be found through the local hospital or public school system.

5. *Recommending, advising, and counseling:* This includes advising and counseling patients and families about the diagnostic results and possible treatment plans. The impact of a particular diagnosis for a child or adult with a communication disorder can be diffi-

cult for parents or caregivers to hear. For families who do not speak English, it is advisable to utilize an interpreter, or a professional who speaks their language. This is where informational counseling comes into play. The ability to tolerate "clinical silence" has been emphasized throughout the literature. In this country, most people feel uncomfortable with silence during conversations. It often has a negative connotation or indicates anxiety or tension on the part of the speakers. In contrast, for individuals in other ethnic or cultural groups (Asian, Native American, Middle Eastern), silence is seen as appropriate and positive (Battle, 1997). Therefore, one of the most powerful techniques for maintaining a client-centered focus is for the SLP to permit and tolerate silence during the interview (Capuzzi & Gross, 2003). Refer back to the guidelines in Chapter 10 regarding this type of counseling.

6. *Treating:* Explanations of possible treatment options should, if at all possible, be in the patient's native language, whether through a bilingual SLP, or an interpreter. It is advantageous to provide non-English-speaking patients or caregivers with written information in their native language describing as many details as possible regarding the treatment plan. Also, once the treatment begins, the SLP should be aware of cultural differences regarding communication styles.

7. *Discharging:* When terminating the therapeutic relationship, the SLP may provide the patient, caregivers, or parents with recommendations for a home program or other follow-up. This, again, should be explained through an interpreter, or someone who speaks

the patient's native language. If other recommendations are made, the SLP should be aware that the family of the patient may not follow through due to cultural differences.

Whether in the university clinic, the public schools, or a medical setting, graduate students in speech-language pathology will be introduced to and gain experience in all of the components of the "cycle of activities." Some health care professions require more cross-cultural competence than others. Specialists in communication sciences and disorders require a greater degree of cross-cultural competence than some other professionals, who see patients for one visit with little need for extensive follow-up. Speech-language pathologists, however, assess and remediate patients' communication abilities, which are deeply rooted in their native cultures (Johnson, 2012).

In closing, we felt it was important to include ASHA's position statement regarding cultural competence as stated in Horton-Ikard and Munoz (2010). This document was developed to provide guidance to ASHA members and certificate holders as they provide ethically appropriate services to all populations, while recognizing their own cultural/linguistic background, and that of their clients or patients:

■ Certain materials may be inappropriate and even offensive to some individuals.

■ Families may choose complementary and alternative medicine, traditional healing practices, and different communication styles, as opposed to mainstream diagnostic and therapeutic approaches. The clinician must have the cultural competence to accommodate these needs and choices, or at a minimum know when and where to seek assistance.

- The clinician must be aware that "differences" do not imply "deficiencies."

- When a clinician is not proficient in the language used by the client and family, a suitable interpreter should be used. The use of interpreters and others who are proficient in the language of the client and family does not negate the ultimate responsibility of the clinician in diagnosing and/or treating the client/patient.

- A clinician must remember that bilingual skill (understanding and speaking the language) does not equate to bicultural skill (understanding and respecting the culture)—both are necessary for culturally competent service delivery.

- Beliefs and values unique to the individual clinician-client encounter must be understood, protected, and respected. Care must be taken not to make assumptions about individuals based upon their particular culture, ethnicity, language, or life experiences that could lead to misdiagnosis or improper treatment of the client/patient.

- Providers must enter into the relationship with awareness, knowledge, and skills about their own culture and cultural biases.

- To address the unique, individual characteristics and cultural background of clients and their families, providers should be prepared to be open and flexible in the selection, administration, and interpretation of diagnostic and/or treatment regimens.

- When cultural or linguistic differences may negatively influence outcomes, referral to or collaboration with others with needed knowledge, skills, and/or experience is indicated.

In summary, speech-language pathologists must develop cross-cultural competence in order to provide relevant interventions for patients and their families as part of serving a diverse population across the life span. Becoming competent in our profession demands that we not only be knowledgeable of racial, ethnic, and/or linguistic differences and their effects on service delivery, but also responsive to the needs of our diverse patient population.

13

Interacting With Supervisors

Communication takes many forms in our field including written, electronic, group discussion, and individual conversation. The importance of one-on-one conversation cannot be overemphasized. We do it with colleagues, supervisors, clients, other professionals, parents, and family members. Part of professional communication is learning how to address these various constituencies in conversational interactions. In some cases, we have these conversations just as a social interchange. At other times, the conversation has a distinct goal such as persuasion, motivation, justification, or counseling. In the previous three chapters we discussed professional verbal communication with clients/families, individuals from diverse backgrounds, and with professionals from other disciplines. We addressed some of the problems that arise and how professional verbal communication can be used to resolve them. This chapter deals with verbal communication that takes place between supervisors and student clinicians. As you will learn during your training, the first clinical supervisors you will encounter are in the university speech and hearing clinic. As you progress in your program you

will no doubt be sent off campus to schools, hospitals, rehabilitation centers, community clinics, private practices, and long-term care facilities. In each of these work settings you will be under the direction of a clinical supervisor. As mentioned in Chapter 2, there are distinct differences between the university clinic and these other settings. The communication issues and student mistakes mentioned in this chapter can occur in any practicum setting, so we remind students to be proactive and maintain an open line of professional communication with your supervisors. Although the information generally applies to all practicum settings, we want to remind you that once you leave the university clinic, everything moves faster. You will be seeing more clients, the schedule will be more hectic, the paperwork deadlines are shorter, and there is less tolerance for practicum student mistakes. These differences are, in large part, due to the fact that you are now working in a facility or school system where professional service delivery is expected and demanded. In the university clinic, everyone knows that it is a training program and the therapy is conducted by students under supervision.

In a hospital, school, or rehabilitation facility, most of the service providers are certified professionals and students are in the minority. Also, your supervisor will not have 20 different practicum students on whom to focus. Therefore, it is possible that you will receive increased supervisory attention as compared to your experiences at the university clinic.

Interestingly, practicum students often report two different scenarios in off-campus settings. The first situation involves a more intensive supervisor-student relationship. This is the product of (a) more clients seen by the same student and supervisor and (b) fewer students to deal with on the part of the supervisor. The result is more time together talking about cases. Because the supervisor has only one or two students to supervise, more time can be spent scrutinizing your behavior. The second scenario reported by students at off-campus sites is less time available for supervisory conferencing. Because the supervisor is busy seeing clients and going to meetings, there is less time for supervisory conferences and, thus, less direction for the student. Some students liken this to being thrown into a swimming pool and told, "Now, learn to swim!" They report less time for the supervisor to explain and model techniques and elaborate on the required paperwork.

Either of the above scenarios can be disconcerting to a practicum student, but take our word for it, the student does learn in either one. In off-campus clinical environments, you will no doubt feel more stress than you did in the sheltered environment of the university clinic, and this stress leads to unique problems between supervisors and students. But we are getting ahead of our story. First, we talk about the nature of the relationship between a practicum student and a clinical supervisor.

The Evolution of Student and Supervisor Relationship Through the Practicum Experience

Whether you know it or not, training programs are designed in such a way as to generate particular expectations on the part of students and supervisors. These expectations change in a predictable way as the student progresses through practicum. Anderson (1988) suggested a continuum of supervision showing that supervision is adapted to the situation and needs of the supervisee. As participation by the student increases, the degree of involvement by the supervisor decreases. The aim, of course, is to develop independent clinicians who are capable of self-supervision. Our own version of this relationship is shown in Figure 13–1, which depicts this change as the lesson of the linking triangles. The triangle on the left with the dotted outline represents the clinical supervisor. The triangle on the right with the solid line represents the student. The height of each triangle represents the amount of clinical responsibility allocated to supervisor and student as time progresses in the training program. So you can see that the supervisor has a lot of clinical responsibility at the beginning of your undergraduate program as indicated by the height of the arrow indicating clinical responsibility. Note that as time goes on, the supervisor's triangle starts to narrow in terms of clinical responsibility. At the end of your graduate program, the supervisor's triangle has come to a point and indicates almost no clinical responsibility. Now look at the student triangle. The student starts the training program with very little clinical responsibility as shown by the pointed end of the triangle. As the students make their way through the program, the student tri-

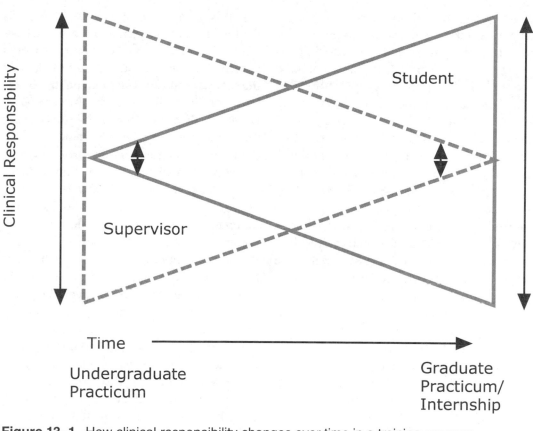

Figure 13–1. How clinical responsibility changes over time in a training program.

angle begins to broaden until at the end of graduate school the student is taking most of the clinical responsibility. The triangles of the supervisor and student are exactly opposite of one another as time goes by.

This phenomenon of student practicum experience suggests that you change as you progress through your training. As a beginning student you know little practical application of your classroom materials, and with experience you become more adept at planning, executing, and reporting clinical activities. This is a natural progression for students as they become more professional and competent. The lesson here is that you should not expect to be the same in your clinical abilities at the end of your graduate program as you were as a beginning practicum student. The transformation of a student from novice to competent clinician also holds a lesson for clinical supervisors. It is unquestionable that supervisors have a sliding scale of expectations when dealing with students in training. For instance, a supervisor has much lower expectations of a beginning undergraduate student as compared to a last-semester graduate student. It is only logical that expectations and grading criteria change over time in a training program. Thus, if you continue to behave as a beginning undergraduate student in terms of taking clinical responsibility, your clinical practicum grade will suffer as time goes by. The expectation is that you will profit from your classroom work and practicum experiences to become more self-reliant and take more clinical responsibility for your cases.

Sometimes a source of difficulty between students and supervisors is a mismatch of expectations between the two individuals. For example, your supervisor may be expecting you to take more clinical responsibility as you approach your third semester in practicum, and you might still feel the need for more help and direction by your supervisor. This mismatch can result in frustration for both parties and a lower grade in practicum for the student. Remember, during your clinical evolution, the expectations of supervisors steadily increase based on your past practicum experience. You will know that such a mismatch in expectations has occurred when a supervisor asks you for rationales, to independently plan a session, or to research your classroom notes for hints on how to handle your client. Another symptom of the mismatch is when a supervisor laments having to "spoon-feed" you as a practicum student. This is your cue to actively take more clinical responsibility and come to planning sessions with your own ideas instead of waiting to be directed by your supervisor.

The Supervisory Relationship

The relationship between the practicum student, clinical supervisor, and client is a unique blend of service delivery, clinical teaching, and student learning. Although the major goal must be the clinical progress and welfare of the client, this is also used as a teaching-learning experience between supervisor and student. In an ideal relationship, the client makes optimal progress, the supervisor can accomplish teaching goals for the student, and the student learns the targeted clinical skills. Sometimes it works exactly this way, but other times there is an imbalance. You can well imagine that this is a very difficult balancing act. The supervisor is not simply doing therapy by proxy using the student as a delivery system. The student is not a neutral conduit through which the supervisor dispenses treatment to the client. True, the student delivers the therapy and learns the critical skills of listening, motivating, taking data, and interpersonal communication abilities with clients. But the student training goal goes beyond the face-to-face skills that occur in the treatment room. In supervisory conferences, the practicum student must learn to understand *why* the treatment goals were selected, how they were arranged in the appropriate sequence, and the proper way to facilitate a session.

Even after all of this preparation, an unavoidable part of clinical practicum is that the student will still make errors in judgment and behavior. Making mistakes and problem solving how to correct them is a valuable part of the learning process. If the goal of a university clinic or practicum setting was simply to do the best therapy for the client, the supervisor would provide the treatment. Clearly, in a practicum experience, there are treatment goals that benefit the client and teaching-learning goals that benefit the student. Obviously, student mistakes can have a negative effect on client progress, so the supervisor must do something to compensate for this. In most cases, the supervisor helps to ensure that the student attacks the client's problem with the very best plan possible. Supervisors do not have the luxury of letting students come up with plans that are not optimal for the client merely to further the cause of student learning. Thus, the supervisor helps the student to generate a sound therapeutic procedure and to understand how and why that procedure was developed. This is done in a supervisory conference through professional verbal communication. Another way that the supervisor "levels the playing field" for the client is to physically supervise many of the treatment sessions or demonstrate specific therapy techniques to make sure the student is carrying out the plan optimally. Typically, less experienced students are supervised more intensively than more experienced students. Although ASHA requires that sessions are supervised a minimum of 25% of the time, most supervisors provide as much oversight as needed, depending on the capabilities of the student and the complexity of the client's disorder.

Goals of Supervisors and Students

The ASHA Committee on Supervision (1985) outlined a number of tasks that supervisors might be expected to perform during practicum experiences with students. Hegde and Davis (2010) explain each of these tasks in more detail, and students are referred to this source for a more descriptive summary. We only list the tasks expected to be performed by supervisors and students to provide you with an overview. Most of the tasks are relatively self-explanatory. First, we can expect clinical supervisors to perform the following:

1. Establishing and maintaining an effective working relationship with the supervisee
2. Assisting the supervisee in developing clinical goals and objectives
3. Assisting the supervisee in developing and refining assessment skills
4. Assisting the supervisee in developing and refining clinical management skills

5. Demonstrating for and participating with the supervisee in the clinical process
6. Assisting the supervisee in observing and analyzing assessment and treatment sessions
7. Assisting the supervisee in the development and maintenance of clinical and supervisory records
8. Interacting with the supervisee in planning, executing, and analyzing supervisory conferences
9. Assisting the supervisee in evaluation of clinical performance
10. Assisting the supervisee in developing skills of verbal reporting, writing, and editing
11. Sharing information regarding ethical, legal, regulatory, and reimbursement aspects of the profession
12. Modeling and facilitating professional conduct
13. Demonstrating research skills in the clinical or supervisor process

Similarly, Hegde and Davis (2010) discuss a number of expectations that a supervisor might have of practicum students. Practicum students should demonstrate the following:

- Compliance with the Code of Ethics of the American Speech-Language-Hearing Association
- Knowledge of ASHA's preferred practice patterns and scope of practice
- Knowledge of and conformity to the clinic's policies and procedures
- Assurance of client confidentiality
- Appreciation of the cultural and personal background of the client
- Evidence planning and preparation for every treatment or assessment session
- Knowledge of appropriate diagnostic and treatment methods in terms

of test instruments and therapy approaches

■ Demonstration of an ability to develop appropriate goals for assessment and treatment sessions

■ Demonstration of the ability to be punctual with both written assignments and supervisory conferences

■ Maintenance of accurate and appropriate clinical records

■ Ability to apply coursework information to the client and engage in appropriate library research when existing information is not available from classes

■ Demonstration of the ability to ask appropriate questions of the supervisor in order to use this mentor as a clinical resource

■ Exhibition of the ability to engage in self-evaluation of clinical skills

■ Demonstration of punctual and regular attendance to assessment/ treatment sessions

■ Ability to accurately maintain records of clinical clock hours and information for certification forms such as Knowledge and Skill Assessment (KASA) documents

■ Demonstration of the ability to act, talk, and write in a professional manner

■ Maintenance of open lines of communication with the clinical supervisor and reporting of any concerns or significant events in a timely manner

It is easy to see that the goals of supervisors and students overlap significantly. For instance, the supervisor wants to show the student how to develop effective assessment/treatment strategies, and this is one of the student's goals as well. From reading the above bullet points you can see that the relationship between supervisor and practicum student is no mystery. We are well aware of the supervisory goals and the learning objectives of the student. However, sometimes putting the teaching and learning goals together creates some difficulties.

Critical Differences Between Students and Supervisors

Clinical supervisors and practicum students typically differ in at least three important ways. Some of these differences can cause misperceptions or miscommunications and make the accomplishment of the above-mentioned supervisor and student goals more difficult. Let us compare the clinical supervisor and practicum student:

1. **Credentials, experience, and perspective:** The supervisor is usually older than most practicum students and may represent the worldview of a more mature individual. Additionally, with age comes attainment of advanced degrees, certification, and licensure. Being a bit older than the student also has allowed for the accumulation of years of clinical and supervision experience. Clearly, the supervisor is operating from quite a different perspective than a beginning practicum student, simply based on age, training, and experience. In the case of the student, he has little professional experience and fewer degrees and has only begun to embark on career training. There is a large gulf between these individuals that can be difficult to span without mutual respect, effort, and professional verbal communication.

2. **Workload:** The supervisor in the university setting is responsible for a case-

load of perhaps 20 to 30 clients, and this probably means 20 different students to supervise. Each of these students has a different level of classroom training and clinical experience, so each supervisory conference must be "recalibrated" to account for these variables. An early undergraduate clinician, on the other hand, may have only one or two cases to focus on. Think of the difference between the supervisor and student just in terms of the caseload size with its attendant differences in clients, student capabilities, different personalities, disparate goals, and varying schedules. It is no wonder that supervisors have a hectic schedule as they move between observation rooms to supervisory conferences to doing paperwork. In many cases these clinical faculty manage to find time to do research and professional projects as well. It is probably true that the clinical supervisor has a much more complicated schedule than the student even when you count the student's class time.

3. **Teacher-student relationship:** Sometimes students beginning practicum forget that the clinical supervisor assumes the role of teacher as much as a professor who stands in front of a classroom. There are some practical differences that reinforce this misconception. First, clinical supervision is usually done on an individual teacher-student basis, and there is no classroom full of students. Second, we usually meet one-on-one in an office instead of a classroom. Third, because of these individual meetings between supervisor and student, there is more of an opportunity to get to know each other as people, unlike the anonymity of the classroom. We raise these differences because they often lead to misconceptions on the part

of students beginning the practicum experience. The first misconception is that the practicum does not involve the relationship between a student and a teacher. However, the practicum relationship *is* a teaching-learning experience just like the classroom, except it is highly individualized and very intensive. In a supervisory conference, there is no way to avoid answering a question like you can in the classroom. There is no way to disguise the fact that you are unprepared. Because you cannot hide, you might feel that you can get by on your personal magnetism and scintillating personality. Some students and supervisors may not want to acknowledge the real nature of this relationship and thus cultivate a "friendly" style of interacting. But, no matter how friendly you become with your clinical supervisor, the relationship is always one between a teacher and a student.

Unfortunately, there is always a somewhat adversarial component to a relationship in which one person is in a position to evaluate the performance of another and assign a grade at the end of the semester. The supervisor has the goal of teaching clinical and professional skills, and you the student should have the objective of learning them. Ultimately, the supervisor will have to make judgments about your clinical abilities, professionalism, and how you are progressing toward independence in your practicum experiences. These judgments must be made no matter how cordial the relationship between supervisor and student. Thus, it is a good policy to make your interactions as pleasant and friendly as possible, but at the same time, you must make meaningful and professional contributions to the teaching-learning relationship. Another common mistake made by students is that they sometimes think that there is no homework involved in clinical practicum because it is not a class per se. Again, this idea is a misconception that could lead the student to lower grades and a less than optimal learning experience. Practicum students are expected to "bring something to the table" from their coursework and prior clinical experiences. The supervisor will expect you to go back to your class notes and look up information relevant to your case. Sometimes you will be expected to read articles and book chapters to prepare for clinical work. Obviously, there is a lot of outside work involved in devising clinical materials, keeping track of client data, and writing goals and objectives.

The three areas discussed above can lead to miscommunication on the part of both supervisors and students. Professional verbal communication is necessary to resolve these difficulties.

Remember the Principles of Professional Verbal Communication

As in professional verbal communication with clients, families, and other professionals, it is important to remember the critical variables of showing respect, being organized, using professional terms, listening and understanding, and paying attention to communicative context. All of these attributes are crucial in dealing with your supervisors. You obviously want to show *respect* for your clinical supervisor because he is experienced, certified, licensed, and in the position of providing you with feedback as well as a grade. *Organization* is important when dealing with supervisors. Typically, there is only a limited amount of time available for a supervisory conference.

You should prepare for these conferences just as you prepare for classes or treatment sessions. For example, you might have specific questions for your supervisor and these should be organized in a logical manner. You should also make sure that the questions you ask cannot be answered by examining your class notes or querying some other source. Your supervisor will be using *professional terminology* in conferences, and you should be prepared to do the same. Finally, you must *attend to the communicative context*. When you have a conversation with your supervisor, you should attend to content and affect, just as we suggested in communicating with clients or other professionals. Your supervisor might communicate frustration by using intonation, body language, or facial expression rather than words. For instance, your supervisor might say, "Didn't you cover this information in your articulation disorders class?" This could mean that the supervisor wishes you had read your class notes on a particular treatment approach so it would not have to be explained to you in a conference. One of the present authors remembers a student who had a very behaviorally oriented supervisor. The story goes that the student arrived for a supervisory conference without her treatment data from the previous week. The student said, "Oops, I forgot my data." The supervisor replied, "Well, without the treatment data we don't have much to discuss except our opinions, do we? So this conference is over." What is the supervisor's message here? Is it just the literal translation of the supervisor's words that the conference was terminated? Hardly. The unspoken message was clearly received. That clinician reportedly never came to another supervisory conference without her data for the next 2 years, no matter who was supervising. Do not forget the critical components of professional verbal communication.

Communication Issues You May or May Not Encounter

When we ask our students about the things that "stress them out" while taking practicum, there is a cluster of complaints that are recycled semester after semester. Interestingly, communication or miscommunication is at the root of most complaints; and all of these issues can be resolved, or at least made more palatable, by acting professionally and using professional verbal communication. Here are some of the most common issues:

1. **Your supervisor wants you to do things that were not addressed in your coursework:** All students enrolled in practicum experiences will develop a relationship with a clinical supervisor. In most cases, this relationship will be a positive one; however, there may be a mismatch between information learned in academic coursework and the goals/activities that the supervisor recommends. Such a mismatch is guaranteed to make the student feel vulnerable, incompetent, and under stress. For instance, the supervisor might recommend assessment or treatment activities that go beyond what was covered in the academic coursework, and the student has to do extra work to learn about this new approach. An example might be that the clinical faculty member has gone to a recent workshop and learned about a technique that applies to the case that you have been assigned. In this scenario you must read articles and handouts that may not be familiar to you from your academic coursework. One way to look at this is that you have been given a chance to learn about a new technique and try to reconcile it with your existing knowledge.

Although the extra effort might cause stress in the short term, it is a great opportunity to learn a new treatment approach and actually try it out on a real case.

2. **Your supervisor does not allow you to do things that you learned in coursework:** Academic faculty members will sometimes report that students complain that their supervisor will not let them use techniques or approaches learned in coursework. In most cases, this is due to lack of communication between the academic and clinical faculty, and not a supervisor forbidding the use of a particular approach. When the complaining student is queried, "Did you ask your supervisor if you could add phonological awareness goals to the therapy?" the student most often replies in the negative. Most supervisors would be elated if a student suggested an addition to the treatment regimen that was based on research covered in the classroom. Thus, in most cases it is not the supervisor's fault, but the timidity of the student in suggesting additions to the treatment plan. There is nothing wrong with asking to use with your client a technique or strategy that you learned in the classroom. If it is appropriate, the supervisor will probably go along with it, and if it is not appropriate it provides an opportunity for discussion as to why it should not be used with this particular client. Either way, it is a good learning experience. But you will never know without communicating your concern to your supervisor.

3. **You only have your undergraduate training and are assigned a complicated case:** In most instances, this probably will not happen. Very complicated cases should not be given to

a beginning student who has not had the coursework to back up clinical planning. If, however, you are given a complex case, you should expect that supervision will be more intensive. Remember, we said earlier that the main goal of clinical practicum is that the client make progress and not be placed at a disadvantage. No one wants this to happen. If you have a challenging case, be sure to do your part in terms of asking a lot of questions, requesting frequent feedback, and researching issues yourself in addition to the information provided by your supervisor. Again, you must speak up and tell the supervisor that you do not yet feel comfortable with planning the treatment for such a difficult case because you have never had the opportunity before. On the other hand, if you are a graduate student who has worked with many such cases in the past, you have to remember the intersecting triangles in Figure 13–1. In other words, you are expected to know a lot about dealing with cases with which you are more familiar. Also, you have acquired basic clinical skills such as professionalism, problem solving, and researching the literature, which you can apply to any case, regardless of the disorder.

4. **Inadequate supervision:** The American Speech-Language-Hearing Association requires that practicum experiences be supervised according to specific guidelines. For instance, assessments must be supervised in such a way that your supervisor watches 50% of your evaluation. In treatment, the requirement is 25% observation time. These, of course, are minimums, and many cases could easily benefit from 100% supervision if the case is complex and the student clinician is inexperienced. Some students report that they would like more supervision than they are receiving on a particular case, and it frustrates them that their supervisor is not more involved. Certainly, most people would want the most supervision that they possibly could get, but you have to consider workload considerations and the ASHA guidelines. Adequate supervision may not be enough from your perspective, but if it meets ASHA guidelines and your supervisor is comfortable with it, that is the end of the story. Over years of working in university clinics, we have seen many supervisors. Some supervise intensively and exceed ASHA guidelines. A *very few* are the subject of student complaints. For example, some students might say, "She's never around," or "I know she wasn't in the observation room at all this week," or "We only had 10 minutes for our supervisory conference and most of the time she talked about her dog." We are here to tell you that such instances are unacceptable for clinical supervisors and most do their job superbly. If, however, you are not satisfied with the amount or type of supervision you are given, the first step is to bring this up with the supervisor. Lay out your concerns in an organized and respectful fashion. For example, you might say, "I'm concerned that I have not gotten any written or verbal feedback on my performance for the past 3 weeks. We also have missed three supervisory conferences. I know you are busy, but I would appreciate your input so I can learn to be a better clinician." If no change occurs, it is important that you use whatever channels are available in your department to communicate this concern to the clinical director or department chairperson.

5. **Oppressive supervision:** In some cases, the supervisor is so involved in the treatment that the student has difficulty feeling "ownership" of the client. For example, a supervisor may frequently burst into the treatment room and "take over" the activity. Some of this behavior is beneficial under the goal of modeling good clinical skills, and you should be grateful for the opportunity to observe. If, however, it happens too much and on activities that you already feel comfortable with, then you should voice this concern to your supervisor. Another example of a supervisor who is being too aggressive is when you are not able to participate in the goal setting for your client. When your supervisor tells you the goals, prescribes specific activities, outlines how you will keep track of treatment data, and does not allow an opportunity for student input, the learning experience is affected. Earlier, we stated that the student should have the opportunity to engage in problem solving, develop strategies for selecting goals, provide rationales, and have a role in planning. If the supervisor is telling you everything to do, it is essentially the supervisor doing therapy by proxy through the student. This is not an optimal learning experience. The student should be able to request a discussion of the treatment program and let the supervisor provide feedback about the student's ability to plan and execute the program.

6. **Personality conflicts with supervisor:** At its very base, the relationship between a supervisor and a practicum student is an interaction between two people. Although we stated earlier that it is the relationship between a teacher and a student, this does not exclude the fact that two individuals are interacting. Just as a student can have negative feelings toward a classroom teacher or a roommate, it is possible that in the more intensive relationship between the student and supervisor, negative feelings can emerge as well. This is generally no one's fault, but just the inescapable reaction of two people who rub each other the wrong way. It can be very idiosyncratic and unfair. There is little to be done about this complaint because neither the student nor the supervisor is going to change his or her personality. So the most productive way to think about this is that you will have scores of supervisors, bosses, coordinators, teachers, and administrators who will be overseeing your work during your career. Although most of these people will be easy to get along with, there will always be a few who are not a perfect fit. Our best advice is to be philosophical about it and treat it as a learning experience. Getting along with difficult people is a skill that will come in handy for your entire career, whether they are bosses, clients, or coworkers. Try to minimize your contact time, avoid pushing any hot buttons, and be respectful of the person. As long as you perform your obligations as a student clinician in a professional and timely manner, you are doing what is required of a supervisee. (Refer to the section on *Generational Differences* at the end of this chapter for a more detailed description of how students and supervisors differ.)

7. **Differing criteria for clinical writing among supervisors:** A major complaint of students is that various clinical supervisors have different criteria for writing reports. A student can write a report for one supervisor and receive compliments on report-writing ability.

When those same phrases are used in a report for a different supervisor, they are deleted with a red pencil and the student is told the writing is unprofessional. It is true that supervisors have idiosyncratic views of how reports should be written. Although they agree on issues such as format and the use of professional terminology, there will always be unique aspects to what they prefer. The worst thing a student can do is to say, "I wrote it this way for Ms. Smith and she said it was correct." You have to decide, as the old country and western song says, "when to hold 'em and when to fold 'em." Arguing about inconsistencies among supervisors is almost always a losing strategy. The best thing to do is to find out from other students and the clinical records how a particular supervisor has approved writing in the past, and stick with that particular style. After you learn the idiosyncrasies of all your supervisors, you can shift appropriately, and you have had the opportunity to learn many styles of writing. When you graduate, you can develop your own style, which will no doubt be an amalgamation of all your former clinical supervisors with your individual preferences.

8. **Differing criteria for grading among supervisors:** Just as classroom teachers differ in their grading methods, so do clinical supervisors. Students are aware that in some classes, most of the students earn A's and B's. On the other hand, there are classes where A's and B's are rare and there is a preponderance of average or lower grades. It is similar in the grading of clinical practicum, although we would suspect based on our conversations with other university programs that grade inflation is especially prevalent in clinical practicum. Most students assume that they will earn an A or B in clinic, but a C is regarded almost as an F is viewed in classroom courses. We are not certain why this occurs in many programs, but it does. Nonetheless, even within the population of clinical supervisors, there are different grading styles; some are simply harder graders than others. In order to better understand the clinical grading system for an individual supervisor, you can see that it is extremely important to discuss the variables you will be graded on at the outset of the semester. Do not be shy about asking what separates an A student in clinic from one who earns a B or a C. Focus on specific behaviors so that you can put your efforts into earning the grade that you desire. Also, do not underestimate the value of frequent conferences with the supervisor to ask for specific feedback on your performance in terms of a grade. Do not be afraid to ask, "If you had to give me a grade at this point, what would it be?" Also, query your supervisor about specific behaviors you need to change to attain a higher grade. Again, professional verbal communication is critical to resolving this issue.

9. **Supervisory conferences that run over time:** It is easy to lose track of time during supervisory conferences. Sometimes the student asks more questions than usual, or the supervisor needs extra time to explain a clinical technique that will be used in the next therapy session. Whatever the cause of running over the allocated time, this should be avoided if at all possible. Due to schedules, the supervisor has meetings, other cases to watch, or other students with whom to meet. Students have classes that abut with the supervisory conference and run-

ning over in the conference will make the student late for class. This is one reason why we recommended earlier that students become very organized about their questions and issues to raise in the conference setting. Supervisors, too, should be able to use the allocated time efficiently and not run over. If the problem becomes chronic, the supervisor will terminate the conference at the appropriate time and ask the student to become more organized. If the supervisor tends to keep the student late, the student needs to say, "I'm sorry, but I have a class this hour and I don't want to be late."

Mistakes Students Make

1. **Complaining to other students:** One thing students have a tendency to do is voice their frustrations to other students in order to gain empathy and support. In most cases, this merely serves to escalate the frustration and spread it to other students. You can be certain that all you will get from your peers is support, sympathy, and validation of your complaint. The student says, "Ms. Paxton wants me to read *two articles* just to work with my client!" The other students say, "Wow, I can't believe she is doing that to you; we have so much to read for our classes. I'm glad I don't have her this semester." And so it escalates until the whole practicum student population is walking around with stifled outrage. Complaining just for the sake of complaining does not solve anything. Actually, when the supervisor assigned the readings, it should have been clear to the student why they were necessary. If it was not clear, then

the student should ask the supervisor what points in particular should be attended to in the articles and how they will be integrated into the treatment. If you understand the purpose of the readings, and if the explanation makes sense, there is nothing to complain about, unless, of course, you just want to whine, which is not very productive.

2. **Not taking time to clarify how student and supervisor evaluations will be done:** In Chapter 2, we mentioned the importance of discussing grading criteria at the outset of the clinical practicum experience with your supervisor. You should be aware of exactly which clinical behaviors are important, your responsibilities, and how you will be graded. If possible, you should obtain a sample copy of an evaluation/grading form that will actually be used in the grading process. There is no excuse for arriving at the end of the semester and saying, "I didn't know that was important and I was being graded on it." Also, in almost every clinic, students are given the opportunity to evaluate the quality of clinical supervision that occurs during a semester. There is nothing wrong with discussing the behaviors that the supervisor will be "graded" on at the end of the term. If nothing else, it will bring to a conscious level in the minds of both the supervisor and the student what attributes are important in their practicum relationship.

3. **Failure to discuss the issue with the supervisor:** All the talking with students and other faculty members will not resolve a problem between your supervisor and you. It is always the best policy to go to your supervisor first to discuss any issue you are concerned about. This can be done in an organized

and respectful manner, and in most cases the issue will be resolved in a positive way. Instead of wasting time talking to other people, go to your supervisor and say, "I was wondering if I might talk with you about a concern I have." We guarantee you that the supervisor will be "all ears" and engage you in a discussion to resolve your problem. Now, it may not always be resolved the way you would prefer, but at least you have aired the issue and will receive a more detailed explanation of the supervisor's point of view. In the case of reading articles mentioned above, the supervisor might say, "The articles will show you how to do three specific tasks with your client, how to gather treatment data, and provide a good rationale for organizing your treatment plan, which is due next week." You still may not like reading the articles, but you have got to admit, the supervisor has some pretty good reasons to ask you to read them.

4. **Copying written materials from prior reports without thinking:** While in clinical practicum in the university clinic, you will often be assigned to work with a client who received treatment for several previous semesters. This client might also have been supervised by the same clinical faculty member during that time. Some students think that an easy thing to do is to simply copy the recommendations from the last report and turn those into a treatment plan. Sometimes these are copied verbatim from the previous semester's treatment report. There are several problems with this approach. First, the client may have changed since the last semester, especially if there has been a long break between terms. A second problem might be that you have a new supervisor taking over the case who may not agree with the recommendations. A third difficulty is that the information in prior reports might be wrong. We have seen, for example, students copy the same case history information section on a client over and over for a string of semesters. In one particular case, three successive reports written by different students stated that the client had normal hearing, when in fact it had never been screened due to lack of child cooperation in the evaluation. The supervisor never caught the error and signed the reports with the students who perpetuated the mistake. It is difficult to keep up with every detail of a client when you are supervising 20 different people. Also, once something is written down in a report, it tends to be treated as fact. Finally, and most important, if you merely copy a series of recommendations or other report information, you have not really taken the opportunity to think about why goals were recommended or how assessment data were gathered. You have not gone through the process of problem solving but are just copying goals generated by someone else. Remember, part of the practicum experience is designed to help you learn to plan treatment in some principled way. Certainly, you should consider recommendations from the previous semester, but you should try to understand why they were made and come up with new considerations based on your knowledge from classroom work. In some cases, the supervisor may be ready to make some changes in the treatment program, and your suggestions will be a breath of fresh air.

5. **Failure to take initiative:** Most students tend to do what they are told

and not go "the extra mile." One way to really impress your supervisor is to come to a conference with some additional material that you have researched related to your client. This additional effort will be appreciated by most supervisors and show that you have a commitment to the case. Even if the supervisor does not want to incorporate the new material, it is something you might use with other clients, and it has demonstrated that you have initiative.

6. **Failure to progressively assume more clinical responsibility:** As illustrated in Figure 13–1, students should assume more clinical responsibility as they progress in practicum. Most supervisors will know where you are in terms of clinical development just by being aware of the cases you have worked with and the number of semesters of clinic you have completed. A major attribute the supervisor is looking for is your ability to apply your knowledge and previous experience to the current case. So if the student says, "I've worked with two other children at this level of language development. In those cases we developed a program like this (hands program to supervisor). I can modify this program with your input, or if you want to go a different direction, I would be happy to learn a new approach." Notice this shows that the student has ideas based on past experience and is willing to use them, modify them, or take a different direction. It shows confidence, a reasoned approach to the case, and assumption of responsibility.

7. **Not being punctual for meetings and assignment deadlines:** A critical aspect of running *any type of clinical program in any setting* is making sure clinical sessions are started and completed on time and that paperwork deadlines are met. One of the most certain paths to a lower grade is to ignore deadlines and clinic schedules. There is no excuse for this, and if it happens to you it is important to acknowledge your error and try to never let it reoccur.

8. **Indicating that you understand when you do not:** Occasionally in a conference you will be told by your supervisor to incorporate a new task into treatment, but you do not understand what it is, how to do it, or why it is important. Some students in this situation will just nod their heads, scribble down some notes, and never ask for clarification. They hope that talking to other students will clarify the issue or looking through class notes will assist them in understanding. It is almost always a losing strategy to not admit when you are clueless. It is completely appropriate to say, "I was with you until you mentioned incorporating distinctive features into the therapy. Can you explain that a bit more, or tell me exactly where I might read about it before next week?" At least in this case you will get a more detailed explanation or a reference that will help you to design your therapy.

9. **Becoming frustrated with lack of client progress:** Everyone knows when a client is not making progress: the client, the family, the clinician, and the supervisor. Sometimes, the lack of progress goes along with a severe disorder. Other times, it is possible that the treatment approach must be adjusted to result in more progress. If you are seeing your client over and over again, and the treatment data are not showing any progress, then it is absolutely appropriate to ask your supervisor about this issue. You can say, "I've been working with John for 6 weeks now and he has

not made any progress. Is this a typical pattern of response to therapy, or should we be thinking about changing our approach?" Chances are that the supervisor is just as frustrated as the student if the client is not making progress. If it is the case that this profile of client response is expected, the supervisor will tell you. If not, it is a good opportunity to rethink the approach, and the supervisor will appreciate the chance to make adjustments. In this case, the student will be credited with being thoughtful and having initiative.

10. **Taking too much initiative when you are uncertain how to handle the situation:** Every student should be aware of his or her clinical limitations. If you have never done a procedure such as parent counseling, it would be inappropriate for you to engage in this without your supervisor's knowledge and consent. A good way to get into trouble is to come to a supervisory conference and say, "Oh, I counseled the parents on what to do at home for Charlie's stuttering." The supervisor might just indicate that such an occurrence is rather strange because the issue of a home program had never been discussed in conferences, and you have no experience with parent counseling. Always check with your supervisor before you engage in any procedure.

Generational Differences

Popular literature is filled with descriptions of the term *generational differences*, and for good reason. There are distinct differences among individuals based on when they were born, and the political, social, and economic environment in which they have grown up (Table 13–1). To begin our discussion, it is worth mentioning a couple of simple definitions of the word *generation* from the dictionary.

> A group of individuals, most of whom are the same approximate age, having similar ideas, problems, attitudes, and so on.
>
> The term of years, roughly 30 among human beings, accepted as the average period between the birth of parents and the birth of their offspring.

The Millennial Generation, born between 1982 and 1994 (estimate), represents a cohort distinct from their parents of the Baby Boom generation, and their predecessors, Generation X (1961–1981). More than likely, if you are reading this book, you belong to this group. (There may be a few outliers who identify more as members of Generation X, or even the Baby Boomers, depending on their age, and/or birth year. It is our opinion that people should claim the generation whose collective persona most reflects their own life experience.) Millennials have been generally described as optimistic, team-oriented, high-achieving, rule followers. In addition, aptitude test scores for this group have risen across all grade levels, and with the higher aptitude has come a greater pressure to succeed.

It is noteworthy to mention that Millennials are the most racially and ethnically diverse generation in U.S. history. As of 2002, "non-whites and Latinos accounted for 37% of the 20 or under population" (United States Department of Health & Human Services, 2016, p. 1), and interestingly enough, they have been described as more accepting of diversity than past generations.

You may wonder why we are discussing characteristics of the millennial generation —we feel that it is important for students in training to understand that individuals from

Table 13–1. Generational Differences

	Boomers *1946–1964* *50–68 years old*	*Gen X* *1965–1979* *35–49 years old*	*Gen Y* *1980–2000* *14–34 years old*
Influences	Vietnam Civil Rights The Cold War	Latchkey kids TV Recession	Helicopter parents Technology
Values	Hard work Competition Success Equality Change	Education Development Creativity Information	Teamwork Input Reinforcement Technology Diversity
Traits	Ambitious Workaholic	Flexible Individualist	Entitled Confident
Communication	Letterhead	E-mail	Text
Timing	Annual	Current	Instant
Technology	Adapting	Adept	Savvy

different generations have different communication styles, expectations of themselves and others, organizational skill-sets, and work ethic. In many situations, you will be interacting with a supervisor who is much older than you are, and who has a very different way of looking at the world and interacting on a daily basis.

Research has shown that children of the Millennial Generation were encouraged to "befriend" their parents, as well as their parents' friends, and as teens they became comfortable expressing their opinions to adults; therefore, they are not hesitant to challenge authority, assert themselves, or ask for preferential treatment. Empirical studies have also shown that Millennials view strong relationships with supervisors to be a crucial factor in their satisfaction with their role as supervisee. It has been

reported that they expect communication with supervisors to be frequent, positive, and affirming. Now, there is certainly nothing wrong with expecting feedback that is positive and affirming. A good supervisor will always point out the positives about a student's clinical skills before providing any criticism; however, the frequency of that feedback may not be as you expect simply because there is a generational difference between you and your supervisor. Therefore, when communicating with supervisors, it is a good rule of thumb to focus on professionalism, and to express your desire for more or less assistance if your needs are not being met.

In today's society, we are taught that to be successful, we need to be self-confident. Some of the characteristics assigned to the Millennials are that they are self-assured, assertive, and perfectionistic, which, when used constructively, can be very positive attributes. What is important to be aware of, though, is that to members of the older generations, this can sometimes be misconstrued as overconfidence. And if your supervisor perceives you to be overconfident, this could create a number of opportunities for miscommunication and misunderstanding. You do not want your supervisor to think that you have more ambition than skill, or that you already "know it all" and therefore do not need his or her instruction or guidance. If you find that you are a perfectionist, take care that you do not allow this to morph into a fear of failure. It is okay for you to admit that you do not know something, and much better to do so than to seem falsely competent.

Millennials and Technology

According to Myers and Sadaghiani (2010), "Millennials are the first generation to have been born into households with computers and to have grown up surrounded by digital media (p. 231)." It is no surprise that individuals from this generational cohort are more comfortable with new interactive media and technology than are older generations. As a result, you bring to your workplace, or your interaction with supervisors, many advantages and beneficial characteristics and skills related to the use of communication and information technologies (CITs). Popular literature indicates that Millennials "have a strong affinity for computer technology as well as computer mediated communication (CMC), and since there are important differences in values and attitudes between generations, it is possible that CMC may intensify some generational differences" (Myers & Sadaghiani, 2010, p. 231). Your interaction with others in the workplace may also change the way your older superiors perceive and use computer technology. In this regard, you may have the opportunity to contribute in a leadership role, once you finish your graduate training and move on to a work environment. It is important to keep in mind, however, that your desire to create personal content on the Internet is not always shared by individuals from the Baby Boom or even Generation X, and that this creates a significant difference between you and members of an older generation; older cohorts still make up the majority of people in the workforce. In addition, Health Information Portability and Accountability Act (HIPAA) laws prevent you from sharing information about clients in any type of electronic format, and your adherence to these laws should always take precedence over the desire to post information on social media, or share information with peers.

Baby Boomers and Generation X

Now that we have discussed characteristics of Millennials, also known as "Generation Y," we would be remiss in not mentioning the characteristics of the Baby Boom generation and Generation X, which will constitute the majority of your supervisors in the university setting, as well as any off-campus clinical placements, future employers, caregivers, and even clients.

The "Boomers," as they are often referred to, make up approximately 29% of the U.S. population. The oldest members of the Baby Boom generation are now mostly retired, and in less than 15 years, one in five Americans (the youngest members) will be over the age of 65. Those who were born at the end of this generational cohort (1960–1964), however, are still a large part of the workforce and may still embody some general characteristics used to describe this group: focused on hard work, ambitious, competitive, and believers in equality. As a member of the Baby Boom generation, one of the authors can attest to the fact that there are many distinct differences between us and college students. This does not mean that we cannot understand each other, or learn from each other; it simply means that we must take into consideration that we may have different ways of looking at the same issue. As we mention in previous chapters, you should always show respect by communicating clearly and demonstrating that you understand what your communication partner feels is important.

Members of Generation X, the cohort immediately preceding the Millennials, were shaped by many factors. Generation Xers learned independence, autonomy, and self-reliance early in life. They were the first to be described as "latch-key" kids, and often took care of themselves and their siblings. They grew up in a time when divorce was commonplace, and therefore ended up in single-family or blended-family homes. As a result, they have been described as being more accepting of themselves and others, and embracing of diversity. Members of this generational cohort have been described as valuing flexibility and creativity, as well as encouraging of individualism. Keep in mind that if your supervisor is only 10 to 15 years older than you are, their ideals and values may be closer to your own but still influenced by issues that shaped them in their childhood and young adulthood.

As we have outlined in this chapter, professional communication takes many forms with many communication partners. There no doubt are other communication issues and mistakes students can make with practicum supervisors, whether there is a generational gap or not. We have tried to give examples of common ones so the student can be proactive in interactions with clinical supervisors. As you can see, professional verbal communication is the medium by which problems with supervisors are confronted and solved. Armed with this knowledge of differences between students and supervisors, as well as information on generational differences, you will be well equipped with the skills needed to navigate your way through any clinical practicum experience.

Appendices

Sample of a University Clinic Diagnostic Report for Child Client Speech-Language Evaluation

Identifying Information

Name: Mitchell Harris

D.O.B.: 04/06/2003

Age: 13.1

Address: 12 Main Street
 Auburn, AL 36830

D.O.E.: 05/27/2016

Telephone: (334) 345-6789

Parent: Vivian Harris

Clinician: Jerome Hamilton

Diagnosis: Language F80.2

Summary

Mitchell is a 13-year-old male who presents today with a mild language delay and moderate deficits in auditory processing, particularly in the area of memory and recall. He was compliant and engaged during the evaluation session. It is recommended that Mitchell attend therapy two times per week for a 1-hour session to address the aforementioned deficits.

Case History/Background Information

Mitchell Harris is a 13-year-old male who was seen at the Auburn University Speech and Hearing Clinic (AUSHC) on May 27 for a speech and language evaluation. He was accompanied to the evaluation by his mother, Vivian Harris, who served as the primary informant. He was referred following an audiometric evaluation and diagnosis of Auditory Processing Disorder (APD) at AUSHC on April 25, 2015. Mitchell has an unremarkable medical and developmental history, with the exception of chronic ear infections as a toddler. His mother stated that her main concern is that Mitchell is having difficulty "following directions from his teachers," which she feels has affected his grades. She noted that he often mispronounces words, such as "pacifically" for "specifically," and that he substitutes words while reading aloud. In school and at home, he requires increased processing time and numerous repetitions in order to comprehend novel as well as familiar information. Ms. Harris noted that she has thought about using written directions at home in order to increase Mitchell's comprehension and ability to perform a task. Mitchell is in a regular classroom and does not receive additional services or modifications to the academic curriculum. His mother reported that math is an area of strength for Mitchell, while language, spelling, and reading are weaknesses. Mitchell is very social and competes on a variety of athletic teams. He is the middle child, with a younger brother and an older brother. He is not currently taking any medications. Mitchell has not previously received speech or language services.

Voice/Fluency

Based on informal observation, Mitchell exhibited age- and gender-appropriate pitch and voice quality. No episodes of stuttering were observed or reported.

Oral-Peripheral Exam

Based on a cursory examination, the structure and function of the oral mechanism are judged to be within normal limits and adequate for speech production.

Social/Pragmatics

Mitchell demonstrated typical interaction skills with the clinicians and exhibited appropriate eye contact. He was cooperative, attended well to activities, and remained engaged in tasks throughout the session. Mitchell exhibited proper topic maintenance skills and initiated and participated well in conversation.

Articulation

Based on informal assessment, Mitchell's articulation skills are within normal limits for his age and gender; no sound errors were noted during the evaluation. He is judged to be 100% intelligible to familiar and unfamiliar listeners.

Language

Test of Auditory Processing Skill-3 (TAPS-3)

Due to concerns regarding auditory comprehension, the *Test of Auditory Processing Skill-3 (TAPS-3)* was administered. Areas assessed included number memory forward (the ability to retain simple sequences of auditory information), number memory reversed (the ability to retain and manipulate simple sequences of auditory information), word memory (the ability to retain and manipulate simple sequences of auditory information), sentence memory (the ability to retain details in sentences of increasing length and grammatical complexity), auditory comprehension (the ability to understand spoken information), and auditory reasoning (the ability to understand implied meanings, make inferences, or come to logical conclusions given the information in the sentence[s] presented).

continues

Subtest	Raw Score	Scaled Score	Age Equivalent	Rating
Word Discrimination	30	9	7:6	Average
Phonological Segmentation	33	11	12:9	Average
Phonological Blending	9	3	5:6	Below Average
Number Memory Forward	15	7	7:3	Average
Number Memory Reversed	8	5	7:6	Below Average
Word Memory	13	5	5:7	Below Average
Sentence Memory	27	9	11:7	Average
Auditory Comprehension	26	10	12:7	Average
Auditory Reasoning	13	8	9:11	Average

	Sum of Scaled Scores	Index Standard Scores
Phonologic (word discrimination, phonological segmentation, phonological blending)	23	88
Memory (number memory forward, number memory reversed, word memory, sentence memory)	26	83
Cohesion (auditory comprehension, auditory reasoning)	18	95
Overall (all subtests)	67	88

The *TAPS-3* utilizes scaled scores that range from 0 to 20, with 10 being the mean and 7 to 13 indicating performance that is within normal limits. Any score below 7 indicates a deficit in the area tested when compared to age-matched peers. Index Standard Scores have a mean of 100 and a standard deviation of 15; scores between 85 and 115 indicate performance that is within normal limits. Any score below 85 is deemed below average when compared to age-matched peers.

Mitchell's performance indicates scores at or within normal limits on all subtests except phonological blending, number memory reversed, and word memory. He demonstrated the most difficulty with phonological blending and memory tasks. Mitchell's greatest strength is in phonological segmentation. He also demonstrated strengths in cohesion tasks, including auditory comprehension and reasoning. Mitchell's overall standard score for this test is 88, which falls within normal limits; however, his memory index score of 83 is below average.

The Token Test for Children-2

The Token Test for Children-2 (*TTFC-2*) primarily measures a child's comprehension of spoken language for children ages 3:0 to 12:11. There are four parts to the *TTFC-2*. Part 1 requires the child to follow one-step directions using all the tokens available (large and small tokens of various colors—"Touch the large blue circle"). Part 2 requires the child to follow two-step directions using the large tokens ("Touch the white square and the yellow square"). Part 3 requires the child to follow two-step directions using all the tokens ("Touch the large blue square and the small green circle"). Part 4 requires the child to follow complex directions using all the tokens ("Before touching the yellow circle, pick up the red square"). Mitchell's scores were as follows:

Subtest	Raw Score
Part 1	10
Part 2	10
Part 3	7
Part 4	11
Overall	38

Percentile Rank	39
Standard Score	96
Descriptive Rating	Average
Age Equivalent	9:6

The *TTFC-2* yields four types of scores: raw scores, standard scores, percentile ranks, and age equivalents. Raw scores refer to the actual number of correct responses in each subtest. The raw scores are combined to give an overall raw score. The overall raw score is then converted to a standard score to compare Mitchell's performance with other children of equal age. Standard scores indicate the distance of the raw score from the average of children of the same age. A standard score of 100 is considered the exact average for the person's age, with a standard deviation of 15 points.

Mitchell's standard score of 96 is within the average range when compared to his same-age peers. His responses were immediate, and he completed the tasks with ease; however, he had difficulty when the directions became more complex or involved multiple steps. The clinician observed that he consistently transposed the colors red and yellow throughout testing.

continues

The Comprehensive Assessment of Spoken Language

The *Comprehensive Assessment of Spoken Language* (CASL) was administered to assess Mitchell's receptive and expressive language abilities. The core subtests were administered, which included antonyms, grammatical morphemes, sentence comprehension, nonliteral language, and pragmatic judgment. The CASL yields standard scores for each subtest, an overall standard score, percentile rank, normal curve equivalent, and stanine. A standard score of 100 is the mean, with scores from 85 to 115 considered to be within normal limits.

Subtest	Raw Score	Standard Score
Antonyms	40	116
Grammatical Morphemes	20	83
Sentence Comprehension	15	97
Nonliteral Language	25	99
Pragmatic Judgment	53	92

Core Composite Scores	
Sum of Core Standard Scores	487
Standard Score	95
Percentile	37
Normal Curve Equivalent	43
Stanine	4

All of Mitchell's subtest standard scores were within or above normal limits except for the grammatical morpheme score of 83. He demonstrated difficulty in this area, which was presented in the form of analogies. At times, he did not identify the correct word tense to appropriately fulfill the analogies. Mitchell's greatest strength was in antonyms, yielding a standard score of 116. His overall language standard score of 95 places him within normal limits.

Recommendations

It is recommended that Mitchell receive therapy at AUSHC at a frequency of one time a week for 1 hour. Therapy goals should focus on the following:

- Improving word recall
- Phonological blending
- Developing strategies to increase recall and comprehension of multistep directions

Prognosis is judged to be good based on Mitchell's language abilities, compliance, motivation, and high level of family support. It is also recommended that Mitchell be referred to an ophthalmologist for a comprehensive vision test to rule out colorblindness.

_____   _____
Jerome Hamilton, BA   Laura Willis, MCD, CCC/SLP
Graduate Clinician   Clinical Supervisor

APPENDIX B

Sample of a University Clinic Diagnostic Report for Adult Client Speech-Language Evaluation

Identifying Information

Name: James M. Bradley

D.O.B.: 07/15/1961

Spouse: Charlotte Bradley

Address: 580 Main Street
Columbus, GA 31907

D.O.E.: 08/14/2016

Age: 55

Telephone: (334) 222-2244

Clinicians: Judy Jones
Ashley Adams

Diagnosis: Aphasia I69.320
Fluency Disorder F98.5

Summary

James "Jim" Bradley is a 51-year-old male who was referred to the Auburn University Speech and Hearing Clinic for a speech and language evaluation following a left hemisphere cerebrovascular accident (CVA). Results of the evaluation reveal that Mr. Bradley exhibits mild anomic aphasia, indicating that he has mild difficulties with naming and relatively preserved auditory comprehension. He also demonstrates a mild neurogenic stuttering disorder with blocks and part-word repetitions. Although Mr. Bradley exhibits a mild stuttering disorder and a mildly reduced rate, he is judged to be 100% intelligible to unfamiliar and familiar listeners. Mr. Bradley was observed to primarily use sentence fragments to communicate. There appeared to be no deficit with comprehension of concrete information during the evaluation. His vision was reported to be within functional limits; however, the audiometric screening revealed a bilateral mild hearing loss. It should be noted that his wife reported that Mr. Bradley was having a "really good day"; therefore, the results of this evaluation may not be typical of his everyday function. It is recommended that Mr. Bradley enroll in therapy to address speech and language deficits resulting from his CVA.

Case History

Jim Bradley is a 51-year-old male who was referred by his neurologist, Dr. Frank Stanley, for a comprehensive speech and language evaluation. His wife, Charlotte Bradley, accompanied him to the evaluation and supplemented the case history information. Mr. Bradley has a remarkable medical history that includes high blood pressure, smoking, anxiety, alcohol abuse, and clinical depression. He experienced a left hemisphere stroke on June 16, 2015. The most recent medical report from Mr. Bradley's doctor stated that while he is experiencing right hemiparesis, he is able to manage activities of daily living with supervision. His wife reported that since the stroke, Mr. Bradley has had "a hard time remembering his words" and that "he talks slow." She also noted that he stutters, which was not present before the stroke. Mr. Bradley stated that he was most concerned with "getting his words out." Mrs. Bradley reported that when her husband experiences word-finding difficulty, he typically abandons the attempt to communicate. Mr. Bradley denies any symptoms of oral or pharyngeal dysphagia. He reported that his vision is within functional limits when he wears his glasses. Mr. Bradley is currently not working due to the residual effects of the stroke but was previously employed by Steris as a machinist. At this time, he is ambulatory and walks with a cane. Mr. and Mrs. Bradley have three daughters who live at home, ranging from the ages of 13 to 18 years old. Mr. Bradley has received no prior speech therapy services.

Assessment Results

Language

The *Western Aphasia Battery-Revised* (WAB-R) was administered during the evaluation. It is designed to measure a patient's language function following a stroke. Linguistic skills assessed include speech content, fluency, auditory comprehension, repetition, naming, reading, and writing. Nonlinguistic skills (drawing, calculation, block design, and apraxia) were not measured due to fatigue.

Results:

Spontaneous Speech Score: 19/20

During conversation, Mr. Bradley was observed to be able to answer questions accurately and appropriately. He responded in a timely manner to questions; however, mild anomia and blocks and sound prolongations were noted. During picture description, Mr. Bradley was able to state the main details of the picture, but he primarily produced sentence fragments.

Auditory Verbal Comprehension Score: 9.05/10

Mr. Bradley was able to correctly answer all simple to complex yes/no questions with the exception of one complex question. No repetition was required.

Repetition Score: 8.4/10

Mr. Bradley was able to repeat words, phrases, and simple sentences, but he demonstrated difficulty when the sentence length was increased to 10 words due to anomia. No verbal apraxia was observed.

Naming and Word Finding Score: 8.2/10

Mr. Bradley was able to provide an appropriate response to complete a sentence for most trials. Semantic paraphasias were frequently noted.

Aphasia Quotient: 89.3

Based on the above results of the WAB-R, Mr. Bradley exhibits Anomic Aphasia. The aphasia quotient is the summary value of the individual's aphasic deficit. Based on Mr. Bradley's aphasia quotient of 89.3, he exhibits a mild aphasic deficit.

The supplemental test for the WAB-R, which assesses reading and writing, was attempted during the evaluation. The reading portion of the test was completed. The writing portion was attempted but unable to be completed due to fatigue.

continues

Results:

- Total Reading Score: 90/100
- Writing Upon Request: 6/6
- Writing Output: 7/34
- Writing to Dictation: 4.5/10
- Writing Dictated Words: 10/10
- Alphabet: 12.5/12.5

Reading strengths observed:

- Choosing the best word from a choice of four to complete a sentence
- Performing simple one-step commands

Reading weaknesses observed:

- Performing multiple-step commands

Writing strengths observed:

- Writing name and address
- Writing dictated words
- Writing the entire alphabet

Writing weaknesses observed:

- Writing sentences about what is happening in a picture
- Writing a dictated sentence
- Prolonged and significantly increased response for all writing tasks

The results of the supplemental test indicate that Mr. Bradley has a mild reading impairment and a moderate writing impairment.

Articulation

No articulation errors, dysarthria, or verbal apraxia were noted during informal assessment throughout the evaluation. Mr. Bradley's intelligibility was judged to be 100% intelligible to an unfamiliar listener.

Voice/Fluency

Stuttering Severity Instrument-4 (SSI-4): The SSI-4 assesses stuttering severity through evaluation of the frequency and duration of stuttering events as well as assessment of any physical concomitants or secondary behaviors that may accompany the stuttering event. For the assessment, two speaking samples were obtained, one was obtained through informal conversation and the other was obtained by having Mr. Bradley read a passage aloud.

Results:

- Frequency: 14
- Duration: 8
- Physical Concomitants: 2
- Total Overall Score: 24

Frequency is measured using a reading task and a speaking task. The percentage of stuttered syllables is computed, and then converted into a task score. The task score for each speaking task is added together in order to determine the frequency score. The frequency score indicates the frequency of stuttering events in speech. The duration score is measured using the three longest stuttering events in seconds. These are then added together and divided by three to obtain an average duration. The average is then converted to a scaled score. The physical concomitants score is based on observations during reading and speaking samples. The only observed physical concomitant demonstrated by Mr. Bradley was slight tension in his neck during speaking attempts. The results of the scores in these three categories indicate that Mr. Bradley falls within the range of the 24th to 40th percentile rank for adults, which places him in the "Mild" severity range.

Hearing/Vision

Mr. Bradley's hearing was screened by the clinicians in the evaluation room using a portable audiometer. In his right ear, he was able to hear 1000 Hz at 35 dB, 2000 Hz at 30 dB, and 4000 Hz at 40 dB. In his right ear, he was able to hear 1000 Hz at 20 dB, 2000 Hz at 30 dB, and 4000 Hz at 40 dB. The results of the hearing screening indicate that Mr. Bradley has a mild hearing loss in both ears. He responded to speech at normal levels during the evaluation.

Mr. Bradley's vision was reported to be within functional limits, and no visual acuity abnormalities were noted during the evaluation.

Oral Motor Exam

The Oral-Facial Examination Screening was used to examine Mr. Bradley's oral motor functions, including range of motion, strength, and coordination. Facial, lingual, labial, dental, and palatal movements, symmetry, and strength were judged to be within normal limits.

Recommendations/Prognoses

It is recommended that Mr. Bradley enroll in therapy to address speech and language deficits resulting from a left hemisphere CVA. It is also recommended that a comprehensive audiometric evaluation be scheduled to assess Mr. Bradley's hearing abilities.

continues

Appendix B. *continued*

Therapy should focus on the following areas:

1. Establishing use of strategies to decrease disfluencies at the phrase and simple sentence level
2. Written language at the sentence level
3. Reading comprehension at a moderate level of difficulty
4. Complex level expressive tasks to decrease anomia
5. Practice use of circumlocution when necessary
6. Other goals as appropriate per ongoing assessment

Prognosis for decreasing disfluencies, learning compensatory strategies for anomia, and writing at the simple sentence level is good. Positive prognostic indicators include intact cognition, self-awareness for errors, motivation, attention, length of time post-onset, preserved auditory comprehension, and family support.

Madeline Moates, MCD, CCC-SLP
Speech-Language Pathologist

Judy Jones, BS   Ashley Adams, BS
Graduate Clinician   Graduate Clinician

APPENDIX C

Sample of Inpatient Rehab Assessment Report for Speech/Language/Swallowing

*Performed on: 02/04/2016 ▲▼ ▼ 1544 ▲▼ EST

General Inform
Pre/Post Treat
Pain Associate
Precautions
Home Environ
Hearing
Auditory Comp
Expression
Reading Comp
Written Expres
Cognitive-Com
Social Interact
Speech Produ
Speaking Valv
Western Apha
WNSSP
BDAE
BNT
Attention Proc
MoCA
SLUMS
SCATBI
SLP LSVT
Special Tests
Oral-Facial Exa
Swallowing Pr
Swallowing Ex
Swallow Asses
Education Hist
Education
Assessment/C
Cog/Comm/Sv
SLP Long Ter
SLP Short Ter
Plan
Therapy Inten:
Recommendat

Cognitive/Communication/Swallow Functional Status

Comprehension Functional Status
- ○ Complete Independence
- ○ Modified independence
- ○ Standby prompting
- ○ Minimal assist
- ○ Moderate Assist
- ○ Maximal Assist
- ○ Total assist
- ○ Does not occur

Comprehension Mode Functional Status
- ○ Auditory
- ○ Visual

Comprehension Functional Status Detail:

Expression Functional Status
- ○ Complete Independence
- ○ Modified independence
- ○ Standby prompting
- ○ Minimal assist
- ○ Moderate Assist
- ○ Maximal Assist
- ○ Total assist
- ○ Does not occur

Expression Mode Functional Status
- ○ Vocal
- ○ Nonvocal

Expression Functional Status Detail:

Social Interaction Functional Status
- ○ Complete Independence
- ○ Modified independence
- ○ Standby prompting
- ○ Minimal assist
- ○ Moderate Assist
- ○ Maximal Assist
- ○ Total assist
- ○ Does not occur

Social Interaction Functional Status Detail:

Problem Solving Functional Status
- ○ Complete independence
- ○ Modified independence
- ○ Standby prompting
- ○ Minimal assist
- ○ Moderate assist
- ○ Maximal assist
- ○ Total assist
- ○ Does not occur

Appendix C. Sample of Inpatient Rehab Assessment Report for Speech/Language/Swallowing *Source:* Used with permission of HealthSouth Corporation. *continues*

Problem Solving Functional Status Detail:

Memory Functional Status

- ○ Complete Independence
- ○ Modified independence
- ○ Standby prompting
- ○ Minimal assist
- ○ Moderate Assist
- ○ Maximal Assist
- ○ Total assist
- ○ Does not occur

Memory Functional Status Detail:

Swallow Update

Eating Functional Status

- ○ Independent
- ○ Mod I
- ○ Supervision/Setup
- ○ Min Assist
- ○ Mod assist
- ○ Max assist
- ○ Total assist
- ○ Does not occur

Current diet order

No active diet orders available.

Progress towards goals:

Compliance with precautions:

- ○ Yes
- ○ No

Detail:

Appendix C. *continues*

213

Appendix C. *continued*

APPENDIX D

Example of a University Clinic Daily Treatment Plan

Daily Treatment Plan

Clinician: Rachel Smith   **Supervisor:** Haynes

Disorder: Language   **Date:** 09/13/2016

Goals and Procedures

Short-Term Goal 1

The client will produce 30 single words or word approximations in order to request, label, or comment with minimal cues after eight sessions.

Procedure

The clinician and client will engage in a variety of structured play activities using high-interest toys such as farm animals, Mr. Potato Head, and bubbles. The clinician will structure the session to facilitate the client's need to request items or activities of interest. The client will be reinforced by receiving the item or activity he requested.

Cues

1. Verbal cue, "What do you want?"
2. Choice cue
3. Clinician models target response

Short-Term Goal 2

The client will follow one-step commands during structured play activities with minimal cues in 75% of opportunities after four sessions.

Procedure

During structured play, the clinician will prompt the client with questions such as, "Put the cow in the barn," "Put the top on the play-doh," and "Give me the ball." The client will be reinforced with verbal praise.

Cues

1. Repeat the stimulus
2. Clinician models the target response
3. Hand over hand assistance

APPENDIX E

List of Selected Abbreviations Used in School Settings

ADA—*Americans with Disabilities Act*

ADD—Attention Deficit Disorder

ADHD—Attention Deficit Hyperactivity Disorder

APR—Annual Performance Report

ASD—Autism Spectrum Disorders

AT—Assistive Technology

AYP—Adequate Yearly Progress

BD—Behavioral Disorder

BIP—Behavioral Intervention Plan

CEIS—Coordinated Early Intervening Services

CRS—Children's Rehabilitation Services

DB—Deaf-Blindness

DD—Developmental Delay

DIBELS—Dynamic Indicators of Basic Early Literacy Skills

DPH—Due Process Hearing

ED—Emotional Disability

eGAP—Electronic Grant Application Process

EI—Early Intervention

ELL—English Language Learners

ELLP—Early Learning Progress Profile

ESA—Educational Service Agency

ESL—English as a Second Language

ESY—Extended School Year

FAPE—Free Appropriate Public Education

FBA—Functional Behavioral Assessment

GEP—Gifted Education Plan

GT—Gifted and Talented

HI—Hearing Impairment

IAES—Interim Alternative Educational Setting

ID—Intellectual Disability

IEP—Individualized Education Program

IFSP—Individualized Family Service Plan

LEA—Local Education Agency

LEP—Limited English Proficiency

LRE—Least Restrictive Environment

MD—Multiple Disabilities

NCLB—*No Child Left Behind Act of 2001*

OHI—Other Health Impairment

OI—Orthopedic Impairment

O&M—Orientation and Mobility

OSEP—Office of Special Education Programs

OT—Occupational Therapy/Therapist

PBS—Positive Behavioral Supports

PST—Problem-Solving Team

PT—Physical Therapy/Therapist

RTI—Response to Intervention

SLD—Specific Learning Disability

TBI—Traumatic Brain Injury

APPENDIX F

List of Selected Abbreviations Used in Medical Settings

A—Assistance

ADL—Activity of Daily Living

ARDS—Adult Respiratory Distress Syndrome

AX—Assessment

Δ—Change

b.i.d.—Two Times a Day

BP—Blood Pressure

c̄—with

CAD—Coronary Artery Disease

c/o—Complains of

COPD—Chronic Obstructive Pulmonary Disease

CVA—Cerebrovascular Accident

↓—Decreased

DM—Diabetes Mellitus

DNR—Do Not Resuscitate

DVT—Deep Vein Thrombosis

Dx—Diagnosis

GERD—Gastroesophageal Reflux Disease

h/o—History of

H&P—History and Physical Examination

HTN—Hypertension

Hx—History

↑—Increased

ICH—Intracranial hemorrhage

L, lt—Left

Max—Maximum

MBS—Modified Barium Swallow

MCA—Middle Cerebral Artery

Min—Minimum

Mod—Moderate

MRI—Magnetic Resonance Imaging

NG—Nasogastric

NPO—Nothing per Oral

O—Oriented (Ox3)

OMEs—Oral Motor Exercises

PE—Pulmonary Embolism

PEG—Percutaneous Endoscopic Gastrostomy

p.o.—By Mouth

POC—Plan of Care

PRN—Per necessary, or when needed

Pt—Patient

R, rt—Right

R/O—Rule out

ROM—Range of Motion

s̄—Without

SOB—Shortness of Breath

s/p—Status Post

s.s.—Signs/Symptoms

t.i.d.—Three Times Daily

Tx—Therapy

VSA/VFSS—Videofluoroscopic Swallowing Assessment

y/o—Year Old

APPENDIX G

Example of a University Clinic Long-Term Treatment Report

Semester Progress Report

Name: John Gates **Age:** 15

D.O.B.: 01/20/2001 **Address:** 1234 Oak Street

Date of Report: 05/01/2016 Auburn, AL 36830

Phone Number: (334) 123-4567 **Diagnosis:** Childhood Onset Fluency Disorder

Parent: Susan Gates 315.35

Current Background Information

John is a 15-year-old male who has a history of stuttering since early childhood. He will be entering the 10th grade this fall in a regular education classroom. According to his parents, John is a "very good student," makes friends easily, and participates on several sports teams at his school. He has an unremarkable medical history and does not currently take any medications. He was initially evaluated at this clinic on October 1, 2015. According to the *Stuttering Severity Instrument-Fourth Edition* (SSI-4), he exhibits a moderate to severe fluency disorder that has a significant impact on his daily interactions. John was receiving speech therapy through the public schools, but was referred to this clinic for further assessment and treatment.

Current Evaluation Results

Date of Evaluation: April 1, 2015

Assessment Tool: *Stuttering Severity Instrument (SSI-4)*

Scores are as follows:

 Frequency: 12

 Duration: 10

 Physical Concomitants: 10

 Total Score: 32

 Percentile rank: 75%–80%

 Severity rating: Moderate-Severe

Assessment Tool: *Overall Assessment of the Speaker's Experience of Stuttering* (OASES)

 Section I: General Information Impact Score: 3.3 (Mod.-Severe)

 Section II: Your Reactions to Stuttering Impact Score: 4.0 (Severe)

 Section III: Communication in Daily Situations Impact Score: 3.4 (Mod.-Severe)

 Section IV: Quality of Life Impact Score: 3.0 (Mod.-Severe)

 Total Impact Score: 61 (Moderate to Severe)

John reported the most difficulty with talking on the phone, speaking with unfamiliar people, and class presentations.

Goals and Progress

LTG 1: The client will improve fluency from baseline at the conversational level with varied communication partners exhibiting less than 5% disfluencies.

STG 1: The client will utilize a smooth, controlled rate during structured reading tasks with minimal cues and 80% accuracy after four sessions.

| Baseline Data: | Date: 02/07/2015 | 3/12 = 25% |
| Final Data: | Date: 02/28/2015 | 11/15 = 73% |

Materials: Eight- to ten-word sentences from *HELP* workbook

Cues: Clinician models smooth rate; "Remember to smooth out your speech"

Reinforcement: Verbal praise, replay audiotape

John made significant progress during structured reading tasks. He stated that it was easier to use a controlled rate while reading, because he "gets into a rhythm."

STG 2: The client will utilize smooth, controlled speech during structured conversation with a familiar listener with no cues and 80% accuracy.

| Baseline Data: | Date: 02/28/2015 | 52% accuracy |
| Final Data: | Date: 04/18/2015 | 88% accuracy |

Materials: *Life Stories* cards, *Converstation* game, spontaneous conversation with clinician

Cues: Verbal cue (remember to keep your voice turned on)

Reinforcement: Verbal praise, "I like how you said that," "Very smooth speech"

John was able to use the strategy of smooth, controlled speech more often as the semester progressed, although his performance varied a great deal from week to week. He stated that when he was under a lot of stress due to schoolwork and responsibilities with sports, he felt it was more difficult to maintain fluent speech.

STG 3: The client will utilize the *Easy Onset* technique during a structured reading task with no cues and 80% accuracy after six sessions.

| Baseline Data: | Date: 03/14/2015 | 10% accuracy |
| Final Data: | Date: 03/28/2015 | 80% accuracy |

Materials: Short paragraphs from *The Source for Aphasia therapy* workbook

Cues: "Remember to prolong the first sound in the word."

continues

Clinician models technique

Reinforcement: Replay videotape, verbal praise

John did well using Easy Onset, although he stated that he wasn't really comfortable doing it, and that most likely, he won't use this technique outside of the therapy room; therefore, it will not be targeted in future sessions.

STG 4: The client will utilize the *Easy Onset* technique when having difficulty initiating spontaneous speech with no cues and 80% accuracy.

Baseline Data: Date: 03/28/2015   10% accuracy

Final Data: Date: 04/18/2015   75% accuracy

Materials: None

Cues: "It sounded like you had difficulty with the word _____." "Let's try that again."

Clinician models technique

As stated above, John reports that although he is able to have success using Easy Onset, he is not very comfortable using it.

Summary/Recommendations

John made great progress this semester regarding his awareness of moments of disfluency, as well as identifying the strategies that were most helpful for him. Even though he initially reported that his stuttering does not hold him back in any way, he eventually shared with the clinician that he sometimes avoids certain speaking situations such as phone conversations and oral presentations. With increased confidence regarding use of his techniques, John has a more positive attitude regarding his speech and stated that he felt therapy had been very helpful for him. It is recommended that John continue with speech therapy at the A.U. Speech and Hearing clinic at a frequency of one time per week for 60-minute sessions during the fall semester. Treatment goals should focus on the following:

1. Increasing awareness of moments of stuttering and avoidance techniques within the therapy setting
2. Increasing the client's efficiency in using fluency shaping techniques (easy onset, smooth transitions between words and phrases)
3. Improving fluency in unstructured speaking situations
4. Increasing self-monitoring outside of the therapy setting

_____   _____

Embry Burrus, MCD, CCC/SLP   Kathleen Palmer, BS
Clinical Supervisor   Graduate Clinician

APPENDIX H

Examples of Data Sheets

Data Sheet 1

Client: _____

Date: _____

Section 1

STG: _____

PROCEDURE: _____

Trials—Record C or Cue # for each trial

	C— Correct	Cue 1	Cue 2	Cue 3
	/	/	/	/
	%	%	%	%

Section 2

STG: _____

PROCEDURE: _____

Trials—Record C or Cue # for each trial

	C— Correct	Cue 1	Cue 2	Cue 3
	/	/	/	/
	%	%	%	%

Section 3

STG: _____

PROCEDURE: _____

Trials—Record C or Cue # for each trial

	C— Correct	Cue 1	Cue 2	Cue 3
	/	/	/	/
	%	%	%	%

Block 1

Trials—Record C or Cue # for each trial

STG:			
PROCEDURE:			

	C—Correct	Cue 1	Cue 2	Cue 3
	/	/	/	/
	%	%	%	%

Block 2

Trials—Record C or Cue # for each trial

STG:			
PROCEDURE:			

	C—Correct	Cue 1	Cue 2	Cue 3
	/	/	/	/
	%	%	%	%

Block 3

Trials—Record C or Cue # for each trial

STG:			
PROCEDURE:			

	C—Correct	Cue 1	Cue 2	Cue 3
	/	/	/	/
	%	%	%	%

continues

Data Sheet 2

Goal/Activity

Cueing Hierarchy   **Data (Number and Percentage)**

1. _____

No Cues			

2. _____

No Cues			

3. _____

No Cues			

APPENDIX I

Examples of SOAP Notes

Example of SOAP Note 1

Clinician: Elizabeth Cochran   **Date:** 06/22/2016
File #: 60-84-25   **ICD-10 Code:** Aphasia I69.320

SUBJECT	Mrs. Jackson arrived on time with her husband. She was compliant throughout the session and demonstrated genuine effort during all activities. She engaged in basic conversation with the clinician by using single words, neologisms, and occasional gestures to communicate. Assessment was continued to establish functional goals for future sessions.
OBJECTIVE	1. The client will demonstrate functional object use with no cues and 90% accuracy after three sessions. 10/10 = 100% 2. The client will provide a correct response in a sentence completion task with minimal cues and 70% accuracy after five sessions. 1/12 = 8% with phonemic cue 10/12 = 83% with full model 1/12 = 8% with written cue and model 3. The client will name common objects with no cues and 70% accuracy after three sessions. 2/10 = 20% 1/10 = 10% with semantic cues 3/10 = 30% with phonemic cues 2/10 = 20% imitated clinician's model She was unable to imitate "toothbrush" or "paintbrush." 4. The client will match a printed word to a corresponding picture from a field of three with no cues and 80% accuracy after three sessions. 6/6 = 100% 5. The client will match a printed phrase to a corresponding picture from a field of three with minimal cues and 80% accuracy after six sessions. 10/12 = 83% 6. The client will respond to simple general yes/no questions with no cues and 80% accuracy after three sessions. 20/20 = 100%

ASSESSMENT	Mrs. Jackson frequently attempted to respond during the session with vocal approximations, neologisms, and paraphasias. She was rarely able to meaningfully use a true word during unstructured interaction. Her expressive strengths included imitation of the clinician at the single word/phrase level and oral reading. She appeared to understand some simple conversation with cues. Her husband offered suggestions of photographs to be included in a trial AAC book. Mrs. Jackson again exceeded criteria for the reading and auditory comprehension tasks.
PLAN	▧ Increase cues for simple sentence completion task. ▧ Create simple AAC book for trial use at home. ▧ Increase difficulty for reading comprehension to simple sentences. ▧ Increase difficulty of auditory questions to moderate level. ▧ Target receptive ability of following one- to two-step commands. ▧ Discharge goal for functional object use due to exceeding criteria for three consecutive sessions.

continues

Example of SOAP Note 2

Clinician: Jaclyn White   **Date:** 07/15/2016

File #: 12-098-1   **ICD-10 Code:** Articulation: F80.0

                                          Language: F80.2

SUBJECTIVE	Charlie appeared to be tired today; he frequently yawned and placed his head on the table. Ms. Dunn reported that he had missed his morning nap. She also noted that he "did real well with his home program" this week.
OBJECTIVE	1. The client will produce /k/ initial at the word level while naming picture cards with minimal cues and 90% accuracy after three consecutive sessions. 7/10 = 70% Cue 1: 2/10 = 20% Cue 2: 1/10 = 10% 2. The client will name pictures depicting common verbs during joint book reading with the clinician with verbal cues and 90% accuracy after four sessions. 5/10 = 50% Cue 2: 2/10 = 20% Cue 3: 1/10 = 10% 3. The client will produce a minimum of 10 four- to five-word sentences with no cues during 10 minutes of picture description after six sessions. Spontaneous: 3 Cue 1: 6 Cue 2: 8
ASSESSMENT	Charlie continued to produce /t/ for /k/ at times; however, he met criteria with minimal cueing. Placement cues continue to be effective when needed. A new book was introduced to address verbs, and his performance decreased from the previous session. Charlie enjoyed the pictures during the picture description activity since they were related to baseball. He did require significant cueing to include articles.
PLAN	Until mastery for two additional consecutive sessions, STG 1 should continue to be targeted. Due to not meeting criteria for STGs 2 and 3, these goals should be targeted next session, with verbal praise and stickers as reinforcement. The same stimuli should be used for STGs 2 and 3 to determine if accuracy will be increased, and picture cards targeting /k/ should be varied to assess generalization.

APPENDIX J

Examples of Long-Term Graphs

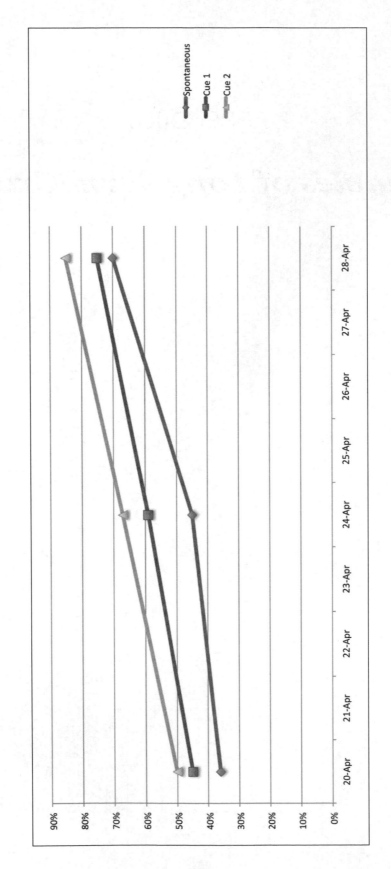

Long-Term Graph

Date	4-Apr	6-Apr	11-Apr	13-Apr	18-Apr	20-Apr	25-Apr	27-Apr	1-May	8-May	10-May	15-May	17-May
100%								*	<	<			*
90%						<	#	*	<	*	#	<	*
80%						<	#	*	*	*	*		
70%	#	#		#		<	#	*					
60%	*	#				*							
50%			*										
40%			*										
30%													
20%													
10%													

cue 1 *
cue 2 ^
cue 3 #

235

References

Alabama State Department of Education. (n.d.). *Mastering the maze.* Retrieved from http://www.alsde.edu

American Academy of Pediatrics. (2007). Professionalism in pediatrics. *Pediatrics, 120*(4), 895–897.

American Speech-Language-Hearing Association (ASHA). (2004). *Evidence-based practice (EBP).* Retrieved from http://www.asha.org/Research/EBP/Introduction-to-Evidence-Based-Practice/

American Speech-Language-Hearing Association (ASHA). (2010). *Code of ethics* [Ethics]. Retrieved from http://www.asha.org/policy

American Speech-Language Hearing Association (ASHA). (2016). *Scope of practice in speech-language pathology.* Rockville, MD: Author.

American Speech-Language Hearing Association, ASHA Committee on Supervision. (1985). Clinical supervision in speech-language pathology. *ASHA, 27,* 57–60.

Anderson, J. (1988). *The supervisory process in speech-language pathology and audiology.* Austin, TX: Pro-Ed.

Atkins, C. P. (2007). Graduate SLP/Aud clinicians on counseling: Self-perceptions and awareness of boundaries. *Contemporary Issues in Communication Science and Disorders, 34,* 4–11.

Battle, D. (1997). Multicultural considerations in counseling communicatively disordered persons and their families. In T. Crowe (Ed.), *Applications of counseling in speech-language pathology and audiology* (pp. 118–144). Baltimore, MD: Williams & Wilkins.

Battle, D. (2002). *Communication disorders in multicultural populations.* Boston, MA: Butterworth-Heinemann.

Boone, D., McFarlane, S., Von Berg, S., & Zraick, R. (2014). *The voice and voice therapy* (9th ed.). Needham Heights, MA: Allyn & Bacon.

Brehm, B., Breen, P., Brown, B., Long, L., Smith, R., Wall, A., & Warren, N. S. (2006). An interdisciplinary approach to introducing professionalism. *American Journal of Pharmaceutical Education, 70*(4), 1–5, Article 81.

Brown, R. (1973). *A first language: The early stages.* Boston, MA: Harvard University Press.

Capuzzi, D., & Gross, D. (2003). *Counseling and psychotherapy.* Columbus, OH: Merrill.

Centers for Medicare and Medicaid Services (CMS). Retrieved from http://www.cms.hhs.gov

Clooman, P., Davis, F., & Burnett, C. (1999). Interdisciplinary education in clinical ethics: A work in progress. *Holistic Nursing Practice, 13,* 9–12.

Cornett, B. (2006). A principal calling: Professionalism and health care services. *Journal of Communication Disorders, 39*(4), 301–309.

Cornett, B. (2006). Clinical documentation in speech-language pathology: Essential information for successful practice. *ASHA Leader, 11,* 8–25.

Council for Exceptional Children (CEC). Retrieved from https://www.cec.sped.org

Crowe, T. (1997). *Applications of counseling in speech-language pathology and audiology.* Baltimore, MD: Williams & Wilkins.

Damico, J. (1987). Addressing language concerns in the schools: The SLP as consultant. *Journal of Childhood Communication Disorders, 11,* 17–40.

Disability & special education acronyms. (n.d.). Retrieved from http://www.parent centerhub.org/repository/acronyms/

Dollaghan, C. (2004, April 13). *Evidence-based practice: Myths and realities.* Retrieved from http://leader.pubs.asha.org/article .aspx?articleid=2292278

Education acronyms. (n.d.). Retrieved from http://www.ncpublicschools.org/acronyms/

Emerick, L. (1969). *The parent interview.* Danville, IL: Interstate.

Family Educational Rights and Privacy Act (FERPA). (n.d.). Retrieved from http:// www.ed.gov/policy/gen/guid/fpco/ferpa/ index.html

Ferguson, M. (1991). Collaborative/consultative service delivery: An introduction. *Language, Speech, and Hearing Services in Schools, 22,* 147.

Fourie, R. J. (2009). Qualitative study of the therapeutic relationship in speech and language therapy: Perspectives of adults with acquired communication and swallowing disorders. *International Journal of Language and Communication Disorders, 44*(6), 979–999.

Fourie, R. J. (2011). *Therapeutic processes for communication disorders: A guide for clinicians and students.* New York, NY: Psychology Press.

Frassinelli, L., Superior, K., & Meyers, J. (1983). A consultation model for speech and language intervention. *Journal of the American Speech-Language-Hearing Association, 25*(11), 25–30.

French, S., & Sim, J. (1993). *Writing: A guide for therapists.* Oxford, UK: Butterworth-Heinemann.

Frequently used education acronyms/terms in special education. (n.d.). Retrieved from http://dpi.wi.gov/sped/about/acronyms

Fujiki, M., & Brinton, B. (1984). Supplementing language therapy: Working with the classroom teachers. *Language, Speech, and Hearing Services in Schools, 15,* 98–109.

Generation. (n.d.). Retrieved from http:// dictionary.reference.com/browse/genera tion?s=t

Generation X. (n.d.). Retrieved from http:// www.valueoptions.com/spotlight_YIW/ gen_x.htm

Gregory, H. (2002). *Stuttering therapy: Rationale and procedures.* Needham Heights, MA: Allyn & Bacon.

Hackney, H., & Cormier, S. (1994). *Counseling strategies and interventions* (4th ed.). Boston, MA: Allyn & Bacon.

Hammer, D., Berger, B., & Beardsley, R. (2003). Student professionalism. *American Journal of Pharmaceutical Education, 67,* 1–29.

Haynes, W., & Hartman, D. (1975). The agony of report writing: A new look at an old problem. *Journal of the National Student Speech and Hearing Association, 3,* 7–15.

Haynes, W., Moran, M., & Pindzola, R. (2006). *Communication disorders in the classroom* (4th ed.). Boston, MA: Jones & Bartlett.

Haynes, W., & Oratio, A. R. (1978). A study of clients' perceptions of therapeutic effectiveness. *Journal of Speech and Hearing Disorders, 43,* 21–33.

Health Information Portability and Accountability Act (HIPAA). (n.d.). Retrieved from http://www.hhs.gov/ocr/hipaa/

Hegde, M., & Davis, D. (2010). *Clinical methods and practicum in speech-language pathology* (5th ed.). San Diego, CA: Singular.

Horton-Ikard, R., & Munoz, M. (2010). Addressing multicultural issues in communication sciences and disorders. *Contemporary Issues in Communication Sciences and Disorders, 37,* 167–173.

Individuals with Disabilities Education Act (IDEA). (2004). *IDEA Part C and Related Topics.* Retrieved from http://www.wright slaw.com/info/ei.index.htm, http://idea.ed .gov/part-c/search/new

Johnson, C. E. (2012). *Auditory rehabilitation: A contemporary issues approach.* Boston, MA: Pearson.

Kaderavek, J. N., Laux, J. M., & Mills, N. H. (2004). A counseling training module for students in speech-language pathology training programs. *Contemporary Issues in Communication Sciences and Disorders, 31,* 153–161.

Klein, H., & Moses, N. (1994). *Intervention planning for children with communication disorders: A guide for clinical practicum and professional practice*. Englewood Cliffs, NJ: Prentice Hall.

Knepflar, K. (1976). Report writing for private practitioners. In R. Battin & D. Fox (Eds.), *Private practice in audiology and speech pathology* (pp. 115–136). New York, NY: Grune and Stratton.

Lemke, A., & Dublinske, S. (2008). Achieving excellence in member service: ASHA's strategic pathway. *ASHA Leader, 13*(1), 20–21.

Locke, J. L. (1980). The inference of speech perception in the phonologically disordered child. Part I. A rationale, some criteria, the conventional tests. *Journal of Speech and Hearing Disorders, 40*, 431–444.

Luterman, D. M. (2001). *Counseling persons with communication disorders and their families* (4th ed.). Austin, TX: Pro-Ed.

Magnotta, O. (1991). Looking beyond tradition. *Language, Speech, and Hearing Services in Schools, 22*, 150–151.

Margolis, R. H. (2004, August 3). Boosting memory with informational counseling: Helping patients understand the nature of disorders and how to manage them. *ASHA Leader, 9*, 10–28.

Marvin, C. (1987). Consultation services: Changing roles for SLPs. *Journal of Childhood Communication Disorders, 11*(1), 1–16.

Matarazzo, J., & Wiens, A. (1972). *The interview: Research on its anatomy and structure*. Chicago, IL: Aldine-Atherton.

McQuire, M., & Lorch, S. (1968). A model for the study of dyadic communication. *Journal of Nervous and Mental Disease, 146*, 221–229.

Mehrabian, A. (1972). *Nonverbal communication*. Chicago, IL: Aldine-Atherton.

Meitus, I. (1991). Clinical report and letter writing. In I. Meitus & B. Weinberg (Eds.), *Diagnosis in speech-language pathology* (pp. 287–307). Boston, MA: Allyn & Bacon.

Middleton, G., Pannbacker, M., Vekovius, G. T., Sanders, K. L., & Pluett, V. (2001). *Report writing for speech-language pathologists*. Upper Saddle River, NJ: Pearson.

Miller, R., & Groher, M. (1990). *Medical speech pathology*. Gaithersburg, MD: Aspen.

Montgomery, J. (1992). Implementing collaborative consultation: Perspectives from the field. *Language, Speech, and Hearing Services in Schools, 23*, 363–364.

Moon-Meyer, S. (2004). *Survival guide for the beginning speech-language clinician*. Austin, TX: Pro-Ed.

Moore, M. (1969). Pathological writing. *ASHA, 11*, 535–538.

Moore-Brown, B. (1991). Moving in the direction of change: Thoughts for administrators and speech-language pathologists. *Language, Speech, and Hearing Services in Schools, 22*, 148–149.

Myers, K., & Sadaghiani, K. (2010). Millennials in the workplace: A communication perspective on millennials' organizational relationships and performance. *Journal of Business Psychology, 25*, 225–238.

National Dissemination Center for Children and Youth with Disabilities. (2008). Retrieved from http://www.nichcy.org

National Institute on Deafness and Other Communication Disorders. (2009). Retrieved from https://www.nidcd.nih.gov/

Neal, E. (2005). *Writing measurable goals and objectives*. Retrieved from http://www.asha.org/uploadedFiles/Writing-Measurable-Goals-and-Objectives.pdf

Nebraska Department of Education. (n.d.). *Setting goals . . . Achieving results*. Retrieved from http://www.education.ne.gov/sped/technicalassist/Setting%20Goals%20Achieving%20Results%203-11-14.pdf

Nelson, K. (1973). Structure and strategy in learning to talk. *Monographs of the Society for Research in Child Development, 38*, 11–56.

Nelson, K. E., Camarata, S. M., Welsh, J., Butkovsky, L., & Camarata, M. (1996). Effects of imitative and conversational recasting treatment on the acquisition of grammar in children with specific language impairment and younger language-normal children.

Journal of Speech and Hearing Research, *39*, 850–859.

Olswang, L. B., & Bain, B. (1994, September). Data collection: Monitoring children's treatment progress. *American Journal of Speech-Language Pathology*, *3*, 55–65.

Owens, R., Metz, D., & Farinella, K., (2010). *Introduction to communication disorders: A life span perspective.* Boston, MA: Allyn & Bacon.

Paul, D. (1994). *Clinical record keeping in speech-language pathology for health care and third-party payers* [updated by A. Hasselkus (2004)]. Retrieved from http://www.dhs.state.mn.us/main/groups/manuals/documents/pub/dhs16_158228.pdf

Paul, R. (2006). *Language disorders from infancy through adolescence* (3rd ed.). St. Louis, MO: Mosby.

Pindzola, R., Plexico, L., & Haynes, W. (2016). *Diagnosis and evaluation in speech pathology* (9th ed.). Upper Saddle River, NJ: Pearson.

Randolph, D. (2003). Evaluating the professional behaviors of entry-level occupational therapy students. *Journal of Allied Health*, *32*, 116–121.

Roseberry-McKibbin, C. (1997). Working with linguistically and culturally diverse clients. In K. Shipley (Ed.), *Interviewing and counseling in communicative disorders: Principles and procedures* (pp. 151–172). Boston, MA: Allyn & Bacon.

Rubin, R. (2014). *AIDET® in the medical practice: More important than ever.* Retrieved from https://www.studergroup.com/resources/news-media/healthcare-publications-resources/insights/november-2014/aidet-in-the-medical-practice-more-important-than

Shipley, K. (1997). *Interviewing and counseling in communicative disorders: Principles and procedures.* Boston, MA: Allyn & Bacon.

Shipley, K., & McAfee, J. (2008). *Assessment in speech-language pathology: A resource manual* (4th ed.). Clifton Park, NY: Delmar Learning.

Smit, A. B., Hand, L., Freilinger, J., Bernthal, J., & Bird, A. (1990). The Iowa articulation norms project and its Nebraska reduplication. *Journal of Speech and Hearing Disorders*, *55*, 779–798.

Stewart, C., & Cash, W. (2010). *Interviewing: Principles and practices* (13th ed.). Columbus, OH: McGraw-Hill.

Stewart, S., & Gonzalez, L. (2002). Serving a diverse population: The role of speech-language pathology professional preparation programs. *Journal of Allied Health*, *31*, 204–213.

Stockman, I. J., Boult, J., & Robinson, G. (2004). *Multicultural issues in academic and clinical education: A cultural mosaic.* Retrieved from http://leader.pubs.asha.org/article.aspx?articleid=2292238

Strunk, W., & White, E. B. (2000). *The elements of style* (4th ed.). Needham Heights, MA: Allyn & Bacon.

Torres, I. (2013, September 10). *Tricks to take the pain out of writing treatment goals.* Retrieved from http://blog.asha.org/2013/09/10/tricks-to-take-the-pain-out-of-writing-treatment-goals/

U.S. Census Bureau. (2011). *Population estimates.* Retrieved from http://www.census.gov/popest/data/national/totals/2011/index.html

U.S. Department of Education. (2000). *A guide to the individualized education plan.* Retrieved from http://www.ed.gov/parents/needs/speced/iepguide/index.html

United States Department of Health & Human Services (2016). Retrieved from http://minorityhealth.hhs.gov/

Van Riper, C., & Emerick, L. (1995). *Speech correction: An introduction to speech pathology and audiology* (9th ed.). Englewood Cliffs, NJ: Prentice Hall.

Wilkinson, T., Wade, W., & Knock, L. (2009). A blueprint to assess professionalism: Results of a systematic review. *Academic Medicine*, *84*(5), 551–558.

Yaruss, S. (2007, November). *Practical treatment strategies for preschool and school-age children who stutter.* Paper presented at the convention of the American Speech-Language-Hearing Association, Boston, MA.

Index

Note: Page numbers in **bold** reference non-text material